YOU ARE NOT BROKEN

Rachael Gilliver

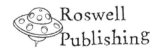
Roswell Publishing

www.raegee.co.uk
Instagram: @RoswellPublishing
Twitter: @VeetuIndustries
facebook.com/thequeenofsteam

Table of Contents

For my friends,
Who inspire me every day with their love for life.

"You are not your illness. You have an individual story to tell. You have a name, a history, a personality. Staying yourself is part of the battle." - Julien Seifter

INTRODUCTION

Mental health still has a stigma attached to it despite advances in medicine and a more open-minded view to the effects of modern life on the brain. At some point in their lives one in four of the world's population will be affected by mental health issues. Yet people still choose to hide, rather than embrace what's happening with their minds, for fear of being ridiculed or accused of lying about their health. Because mental health issues can't be seen people fear what will happen if they stand up and say, "Hey, I have depression/bipolar/PTSD". Some people just don't feel comfortable talking about their minds because, to them, the illness isn't real due to its invisibility.

It's time for the stigma to end and for people to embrace who they really are. It's time for mental health issues to come to the forefront and for people to be proud of who they are. Because it takes a lot of courage to wake up every morning and battle the same demons that left you so tired the night before.

I'm bipolar and I'm proud of it. I've coated this brain of mine in glitter and given it a full on parade. I'm not scared of what it throws at me. Rather I love it for its delightful imperfection. I don't see my bipolar as a problem. Rather I embrace it, dance with it, and let it take me on some inspiring journeys.

However, along the way, I've had to overcome fears. I've had to battle with a mind that won't allow me to travel, create, or leave the house. I've had to beat it down and teach it that whatever it's scared of isn't real.

From 2004 to 2015, I was medicated with a range of different drugs. The final one that I took was a daily of 200 milligrams of Seroquel. Over the course of a year, from April 2014 to April 2015, I was slowly weaned off of it until, in March 2015, I took the final dose.

The drugs turned me in to a zombie and, for me, froze time. For eleven years, I lived in a state of stunted development only to emerge in a world that I didn't recognise or understand. My emotions hadn't had the chance to evolve with me and I had trouble translating what I was feeling.

Luckily I had two psychologist friends who, for the first few months, helped me to learn how to react to the world around me. They're still at the end of the phone if I need them, acting as emotional translators in a frequently bizarre world.

During that time I blogged about what I was feeling as well as how I was dealing with the brave new world around me. Over time I realised that I'd put a lot of useful information on my website and decided that it was time to share it with as many people as possible rather than keeping it to the few people who pass by my blog.

I know that concentration can be hard when your brain isn't as it should be so the chapters in this book have been kept to 500-1000 word, blog size chapters. Often, with mental health, we choose to focus on the brain and why it's acting like it is. We are more than just our brain so this book contains little snippets to help you to heal you mind, body, soul, and spirit. You can read the book from cover to cover or dip in and pick the chapters that are relevant to you.

You Are Not Broken is not intended to ignore or belittle your illnesses or issues. Rather it's a book that will hopefully help you to come out of the mental health closet and be the beautiful person that you are. Within these pages are the tactics that I've used to embrace my brilliant brain and enjoy the ride that it takes me on.

I hope that you have a beautiful, blessed, and brilliant life!
Rae :)

YOU ARE NOT BROKEN

Often, when faced with the issues our brain gives us, we're lead to believe that we're broken. Imperfect. Not "normal". We're lead to believe that we need fixing and that, in refusing help, we are upsetting the status quo. The world wants "normality". It doesn't want broken people. Let me tell you this:

You are not broken.

You are a unique creation. One of a kind. There is only one of you. The mould was broken when you were born. There will never be another one of you. No one will share your unique characteristics. No one will look like you. No one will have your voice or your personality. No one will take the life path that you're taking.

You are not broken.

Mental health is a subject that is often overlooked. It is pushed away. Hidden. An issue that many see as a weakness. To have something wrong with your brain means that you are weak, inferior, or not a part of the human race. But what if you're not supposed to be a normal part of modern society? What if you're supposed to express yourself differently from those around you? What if you're supposed to see the world through different eyes?

You are not broken.

Some people choose to use medication to work with their mental health. This isn't wrong. Some people decide that medication isn't the route for them. This isn't wrong.

Some people go and see a therapist. This isn't wrong. Some people may decide that walking by the sea is their therapy. This isn't wrong. Some people may decide that yoga, meditation, or journaling is the way to go for them. This isn't wrong. Some people may seek solace in religion. This isn't wrong. There is no right or wrong way for a person to deal with what is going on in their brain. Ultimately, it's whatever works for them. The same goes for you; if something is working and making you feel better, keep on doing it.

You are not broken.

You are far from being broken. Your brain is as unique as you. You may find that you work faster and harder than other people. Or that you need to take time out between tasks. Only you know how your body works and you should never let another person dictate to you how you should be leading your life. If something works for you, and it makes you feel comfortable with the person you are, then good for you! You're on your way to beating the battle.

Never forget that you are not broken.

MIND

LIFE AFTER DIAGNOSIS

Firstly, don't panic. While a diagnosis may feel like the end of the world, it's not. Having a diagnosis can be a positive thing.

You now know what's wrong with you. Whatever you have now has a name and a face. You can read up on it and start working on the best course of treatment. You can learn to embrace your diagnosis and love it. And, no matter what anyone tells you, you are not broken.

Secondly, a diagnosis is useful in so many other ways. As well as being able to work on a treatment plan, you can now explain to people why your behaviour might be a little "off" or why you may be having a bad day. Should something happen to you healthcare workers will have a starting point as well as knowing what medications you're taking.

I went through the struggles of not knowing what was wrong with me. My moods wouldn't settle and there were days when I seemed to sleep forever. There is a history of depression in my family so that was where the doctors started.

Following that, I was exhibiting schizophrenic symptoms so that was the next place that the medical team visited.

That was eventually ruled out and the diagnosis of Bipolar Type 2 was settled on. My moods were fluctuating but only very slowly. I spend a lot of time in a stable state and can always tell when my mood is about to change. There's either a slow climb to mania or a slow descent to depression. Because I know the warning signs, I can work on pulling myself back in to a healthy state of mind. If you know what triggers your mental health issues, awesome! If you don't know the triggers, take the time to begin learning them. That way you can have more control over how you look after yourself. You'll also feel better for it.

Learn as much as you can about your diagnosis. Read books and websites, talk to other people, research the medicines you've been given (if you're taking medications) and look in to holistic medicines, too. Even though I'm no longer medicated, I've found that things like massage, relaxation music, and essential oils are perfect for lifting up my mood. You may have things that already work for you. If you don't, have fun experimenting!

Your diagnosis is not a label. Your diagnosis is also not who you are. You don't need to describe yourself as a person with "X illness". You are far more than a label and a medical term. Think of yourself as a human with super powers instead (My super powers include being able to spend long hours concentrating on writing and being able to fall asleep anywhere!).

No matter what you've been through, life after diagnosis can only get better. The days may seem dark at first but they will become lighter. Believe in yourself!

DON'T DWELL ON THE PAST

This chapter came from an email conversation with a friend and reminded me of how we like to live in the past. Sometimes the past was a good place. Sometimes it was a bad place. Sometimes people we loved sadly disappear from our live. Sometimes we wonder what happened to the people we disliked. Sometimes we wonder if we were a better person back then.

We spend a lot of time in the past, analysing ourselves and the relationships that we've had, whether they were with family, friends, or people on the street. We look at how we treated those around us and whether our own boundaries were respected.

The past is a comfortable place to be. It's far less terrifying than whatever the future may hold. But the past is also not the best place to be. Yes, we may learn about the patterns which make us who we are. But it can also keep us locked in a cycle of darkness and depression. The past can fuel our fears and insecurities. It can make us paranoid and fearful of what's to come. There's also a lot of "What if's" in the months and years that have passed us by. We wonder why we didn't take up certain opportunities. We look at the people who were there with us and compare ourselves to their lives. Are they better or worse than us? Do they deserve the life they have? Why can't I have the life that they have?

We'll never know what other peoples lives are like so there's little point in comparing ourselves to them.

Looking to the future and all that it can hold is the way to go.

But it can be hard to let go of the past. Hard to let go of all that we had and all that we experienced. In order to let go of what has been we have to look at what could be. What could you be in a year's time? Where do you want to be twelve months from now? Write it all down and read it out loud to yourself. Make it real in your head. Once you've done that, thank yourself for the past you've had, whether it's been good or bad. Say thank you and begin moving forwards. You can create a life for yourself that doesn't involve weeks and months living the life that has been. Look up and live the life that could be.

THREE IS THE MAGIC NUMBER

There's a saying that everything comes in threes. When the universe sends us signs we tend to see them in threes. The writing rule of three suggests that things coming in threes are funnier, more satisfying, or more effective than other numbers. People are said to remember information better if it's given to them three times.

For this exercise, we're going to work in threes. It's up to you to choose what goes in the lists.

Three Things That You Love About Yourself

1.

2.

3.

Three Things That You Love Doing

1.

2.

3.

Three Things That You'd Love To Do With Your Life

1.

2.

3.

Three People That You Hold Dear To You

1.

2.

3.

Three Places That You'd Love to Travel to

1.

2.

3.

Three Songs That You Love

1.

2.

3.

Three Films That You Love

1.

2.

3.

Three Books That You Love

1.

2.

3.

Three Things That You Would Do If Money Was No Object

1.

2.

3.

Three Dreams That You Have For Your Life

1.

2.

3.

  Once you've written your lists, look them over and think about why you love those things so much. Feel the warmth, love, and excitement that they bring. Whenever you need to remember who you are and why you're in this world, come back and read over them.

  As for the dreams, well, they're yours for the taking. Start working on them!

CHOOSE YOUR THOUGHTS

Choose your thoughts wisely for they can make you feel like heaven, or drag you down to the deepest, darkest depths of your subconscious.

What are you thinking right now? Are you thinking about what goodness your life may bring in the future? Or thinking about that moment two weeks ago when you said the wrong thing at the wrong time? How do the different thoughts make you feel? Do the positive ones makes you feel good? Do the negative ones make you feel like you're walking through mud?

It's true that what we're thinking can affect how we feel. However when you're trying to live with a brain that doesn't always work staying on the positive side of life can be difficult. Often we're dragged down by our thoughts. We spend hours questioning the why's and wherefore's. We wonder how illness could take over our body while our friends are living lives that, to us, look like pure luxury. We curse the person who cut into the line, or who overtook us at the wrong moment, or who said the wrong thing to us. We dwell on them and allow them to become large, swirling dragons in our stomachs. We feel our bodies tighten in response to these thoughts and our heads begin to pound as the anger grows.

Getting past the negative thoughts can seem easy when written down and presented to you as the chapter of a book. But when you live with mental health issues it can be a lot harder. We can spend a few days living with our positive thoughts and thinking that we're back on the right track before the dark days return. Suddenly, in the blink of an eye, we're ready to be pulled back under, cursing at the person who sent us a nasty email or left us an unforgivable comment.

I'm not immune to negative thoughts. Lines at shops; someone walking too slowly in front of me; my phone battery dying. All of them can trigger some kind of negativity and, once it does, I notice other thoughts creeping in. The people who've wronged me in the past; the opportunities that disappeared overnight; why my friends have better lives than I do. When those kinds of thoughts begin to creep in, I pause, and tell them that, no, they're not taking up space in my head. While it may be a struggle, I remind myself why I love my friends. I realise that those missed opportunities may not have been right for me. And I remember that the people who wronged me may have their own problems to deal with.

It's important to recognise when the negative thoughts are happening. Whenever you see or hear something that is likely to trigger the negativity, take a step back and tell yourself that you're not going down that path. You're not going to live with darkness and negativity. Once you've caught yourself focus on the good things that can happen, and are happening, in your life, even if it's just spending a few moments outside in the sunlight. Dwell on that and be thankful for it. Say thank you to the sun. Say thank you to the person who let you cut in line. Say thank you for the food on your plate. When you say, or think, those thankful words you're helping to chase away the negativity.

Over time you'll find that you're more inclined to lean towards positive thinking. Yes, the negative thoughts will still rise but you'll be able to push them back and keep it at bay.

Keep your life as positive as possible and see what a difference a smile instead of a frown can do. Be happy!

WHERE'S YOUR P.M.A.?

(That's Positive Mental Attitude!)

Even during good days, having a positive mental attitude can be hard. How do you keep a happy outlook when the world around us is so dark? How do you spread kindness and love when other people are intent on destroying themselves and the world around them? How can you escape the darkness of your brain when the global outlook is already so bleak.

Creating a positive mental attitude can be hard. It takes time and effort. Like many things, starting small is the way to go. Your attitude won't completely change overnight and, like everything, you are in a constant state of evolution.

I started with a Gratitude Journal when I wanted to change from a negative to a positive way of thinking. At the beginning of the year, I bought a diary and every day I wrote three things that had made me happy that day. They were simple things like receiving something in the mail, or hearing my favourite song, or seeing the sun rise. As the months went by, I found that I was becoming grateful for more things until the list I was writing wouldn't fit on to a single page. Every day I found new things to say thank you for and I noticed that people's attitudes towards me were also changing. Whereas they had once avoided me, I now noticed that complete strangers would smile and open up to me. It was, quite literally, life changing.

I felt lighter and happier in myself and my smile refused to fade. Even now I notice how heavy I feel when I'm in a low mood and negative thoughts are rolling through my brain. But I can pinpoint that it's happening and do something to help lift my mood. This might be going for a walk, reading a book, listening to music, or talking to a friend. For me, having a positive mental attitude has radically helped with the issues that plague my brain.

There's so many ways that you can kick start your own P.M.A. You can keep a Gratitude Journal. You don't have to begin at the start of the year. Grab a diary or blank notebook and jot down the things that make you happy.

Try and enjoy the little things in life; a walk in the park, hearing your favourite song, or dancing (it doesn't matter if you can't dance. Find a quiet spot and go for it! I can't dance but it's still one of my favourite things to do!).

Any creative outlet is good for getting that P.M.A. going, whether it's writing, playing music, or creating art.

While it can be a great tool for keeping in touch, social media can become a hindrance in your life when it comes to positive thinking. Unfollowing negative pages and people is one place to begin. Disconnecting from those people can be really difficult, especially if they're close family or friends. However, most social media sites provide you with both an unfollow and an unfriend button. Use the unfollow button and you'll still remain a part of their digital life therefore bypassing those awkward conversations about why you may have deleted someone from your friends list. Find positive people and pages to follow instead, the ones who post inspiring quotes and uplifting photographs.

Keeping a positive mental attitude can be easy. You just have to choose to start!

BATTLING DEPRESSION

I ache. I ache all over. From my head down to my toes, I ache. I'd forgotten what depression is like. I'd forgotten that it's an all encompassing feeling that swathes you in a cloak of black and forces you to... stop.

I don't want to do anything. I don't want to get up. I don't want to eat. I don't want to drink. I don't want to shower. Even sitting in front of the TV is painful.

I've never been affected by Seasonal Affective Disorder (SAD) before. For 11 years, I was medicated against the effects of the seasons. In fact I never even realised that the changing of the seasons could make you feel happy or sad or somewhere in between. All I knew was that summer followed spring, that autumn followed summer and that winter followed autumn. My mood, through it all, was nice and level and predictably unchanging.

But this winter has been so much different to the previous ones. Now that the medication is well and truly gone, I'm feeling everything that I've never felt before. For the past few weeks I've wanted to do nothing more than cry and sleep. Even keeping my eyes open has been painful at times. My brain doesn't always make the necessary connections, making it hard for me to think properly or even to answer a question correctly. Stress and anxiety have forced my body to tighten to the point of agony and my breathing is so shallow that my ribs now ache from the lack of effort.

I've been lucky in my mental health journey. I never

knew that the winter months could make you feel like this. I never knew that they could be so cripplingly painful. I never knew that there would be days when I'd have to fight, not just to stay awake, but also to retain my sanity.

It's not been an easy few weeks but it's slowly getting better. I've written 25,000 words in the last three weeks so that's made me happy. Watching the days become slowly longer has made me hopeful for the future.

But your brain, like the rest of your body, is a working organ. It does get sick and it's not a bad thing to go to the doctor and get it checked out. You may already know if there's something wrong with your brain. No matter what you have, you can win. You are not bound by what your brain dictates to you. Your thoughts and emotions are all yours, and you're free to change them whenever you please. Battle the negative thoughts with all your might and welcome the positive ones with open arms. Bare your teeth at the darkness and dance with the light. You can live a happy and fruitful life.

MENTAL AEROBICS

Mental patterns are hard to break. You may wake up in the morning and all you can think about is work and the people that you have to interact with. Or you may think you're not good enough. These thoughts go around our head, snowballing in to something far greater than we need. They become like a ball and chain around our ankle, unbreakable and unshakeable.

These patterns happen to everyone and, just when you think you're rid of them, they pop up like that 1990's boy band on a reunion tour. You can't seem to shake them, no matter how hard you try. Often we find ourselves performing complicated mental aerobics just to try and retain some kind of positivity in our lives.

I suffer with these thoughts just like everyone. There are some mornings when I don't want to get up because I'm hot with anger from a conversation I had the day before. Or I have a splitting headache because I've spent several hours dwelling on the wrong assumption that someone has made about me. I'm too fat, too short, too ugly. You name it and I've probably thought it at some point.

Negative thought patterns can be broken. In order to get them out of your life for good, you need to recognise when they're starting to take over your life. At the end of the day, look back and see how you felt at certain moments during the day. If there was a period when you were feeling great, what were you thinking about at that time? What were your thoughts when you were feeling depressed, tired, or elated? What had happened to trigger those thoughts?

Words carry so much power and replacing just one word in a sentence can make all the difference to how you feel. Try some of the examples below and see how the different phrase make you feel. Work with your own to turn them from the negative to the positive.

"I am not good enough." becomes "I am good enough."

"I am sick." becomes "I am well."

"I am broken." becomes "I am whole."

"I am ugly." becomes "I am beautiful."

"I hate myself." becomes "I love myself."

"I am too fat/too thin/too short/too tall." becomes "I am perfect the way I am."

Of course there are times when the negativity that we feel isn't directed at ourselves. Rather its outside influences like managers, family, and co-workers who are the basis for our negative thoughts. There's very little that we can do to change them as a person. But we can change our outlook.

Remember that their stress is not your stress. You are not obligated to take their stress on board and carry it with you. Their anger is also not your anger. Even if you feel like it is, it isn't yours and you can let that go. When you have a quiet moment to yourself, close your eyes, take a deep breath and say, "I let this stress and anger go. It's not mine to carry around and I will not be burdened with someone else's problems.".

Try and limit your access to places that you know trigger the negative thinking. If fashion magazines make you feel hopeless, try to stop buying them. If the news makes you feel hopeless, stop watching the news or at least listen to it in smaller doses. If certain people make you feel depressed, try and limit your time with them.

Being in a negative state isn't a natural state of being. While we have the ability to feel whatever we want to feel, being happy is far better for your health. Be happy and be healthy!

JUDGEMENT

We're all judgemental whether it's of ourselves or other people. We've all stood behind someone who's taking their time in the store, quietly cursing them in holding up our day. We've all looked at ourselves in the mirror and thought that we're too fat, too thin, too tall, too short, too ugly.

We're our own harshest critics in that we can, and will, tear apart everything we do and everything we see. I'm not immune; I'm sitting here, reading every word I write and wondering if this book is the right thing to be doing. To me, my writing seems too simple, too pedestrian. Or the idea's been done before, or I'm not doing it well enough. I've also been behind someone who's taking their time and silently judged them for not having the correct change ready or for asking questions that they should know the answers to.

I have to remind myself that I'm not everyone else and not everyone else is me. We all have different qualities and ways of processing information. Some people may need to ask a lot of questions. Others may be happy to walk in and out of a store without so much as saying a word to another person. As we all know, our brains work very, very differently to one someone else's.

Judgement can be especially harsh within the mental health community. We may deem ourselves too ill or not ill enough. We may find that we look down on others or find that it's us who are being looked down upon.

So how can we prevent judgement? The answer is that we can't, at least not when it's coming from other people. And while we won't be completely clear of it, we can move to change our thinking to a more positive thought form.

One method I've used over the years is to wear a rubber band around one wrist. Whenever I find negative thoughts passing through my mind, I flick the band just hard enough to pull myself back. It's a quick way of pulling your thoughts away from whatever negativity you're focusing on.

Fill your mind with the good that surrounds you. It may be in short supply some days but there is always something to be happy about. A sudden rain storm. A ray of sunlight. A good cup of coffee. Try and focus on the good in other people if you find yourself judging or comparing yourself to others. You don't have to speak to them but mentally compliment their hair, or their shoes, or the outfit they're wearing.

Smile whether you're feeling like it or not. Smiles help to lift the body's spirits, making you feel better and helping those around you to feel the warmth that radiates from you.

Over time you'll feel the negative thoughts begin to fade away. As and when they return, because they will, you'll be prepared for them. And you'll notice just how much different you feel when you've passed up on being judgemental. Judgement carries a weight to it, hanging around our bodies like lead. Being positive, on the other hand, can make you feel as though you're walking on air.

Smile and the world truly will smile with you.

STIGMA

There's still a lot of stigma attached to mental health. Because of the invisibility of the illnesses, people with mental health issues are often challenged on their diagnosis, accused of seeking attention, or told that they're outright lying. For many people, the stigma runs so deep that they feel the need to become Oscar winning actors in order to hide their issues. When you feel like your whole existence is being threatened because of the comments that one person made, it's no wonder so many people refuse to talk about what's going on in their lives.

Mental health needs people like you and I to help end this stigma. Just because something can't be seen doesn't mean that it doesn't exist. We don't dispute the existence of gravity, oxygen, or electricity purely because we can't see them. So why dispute the existence of mental health issues?

We need to open up and talk more. We need to stand up for those who are weaker than ourselves. We need to be the voices of the mental health charities. We need to be the worker bees that help to join up the dots of often frustrating health systems. We need to be the people who campaign for better treatment, better education, better workplaces, and better attitudes. We need to be the ones who put an end to negative comments surrounding mental health issues.

Offer advice. Offer a shoulder to lean on. Offer your time. Offer your own experiences. You are not alone in this world and whatever you've faced can help others to step in to their light. You can help them to open their doors and be free of prejudice and judgement. You can help them feel loved, wanted, and needed in a world that may have shunned them.

Your contribution to the world may feel small. But starting a blog, a Twitter account, or Facebook page can be as powerful as a person who speaks from a stage. What matters is that you're putting your voice out there and helping to break the stigma that holds so many people prisoner.

If you feel scared and alone, reach in to the darkness and find a hand to grasp. It may be a friend, a co-worker, or a complete stranger. But someone will pull you up and give you the courage and confidence to stand up and be counted.

Along the way, you will find people who will love you as much as you love those around you. People will care for one another, making sure that you, in your campaign for a better world, are also looked after. Everything goes around in circles and as you put your love and light in to the world, so it will be returned to you by others. Take care of each other. Lift one another up. Hug each other when the going gets tough and celebrate when you have a breakthrough. Most of all, help to end the stigma that comes with mental health.

You are not alone and you are not broken. You are a wonderful and unique creation who has a story to tell the world, a story that will help others to also heal themselves.

PICK ME UP

When you're feeling down, what do you do to make yourself feel better?

At the moment, my apartment smells of lemongrass. Tea-lights flicker in the oil burners and the light, citrus smell instantly lifts my mood. Whenever I'm feeling low I revisit some of my favourite places be they books, songs, films, memories, or physical locations. I let my mind wander and think of the places I'd like to see and the people I'd like to meet.

Essential oils are a perfect and natural way to lift your mood. Add a few drops to an oil burner or vaporiser. You may already have favourites of your own. If not, good oils to start with include:

- Lemongrass
- Peppermint
- Cinnamon
- Lavender
- Chamomile
- Lemon

Chocolate, as many of us probably already know, is a great mood lifter. This is because chocolate releases that wonderful happy hormone, Serotonin. So never feel guilty for having that chocolate because it really is helping you to feel better.

It's not a lie; studies are showing that a cat's purr can

apparently heal. Their constant pattern of purring resonates between 25 and 150 Hertz which, for the cat, are the frequencies that help to relax muscles and tendons and improve bone density. But that soft soothing sound also helps us. Having a pet close by has been shown to lower stress and reduce depression. If you have a cat, cuddle them often as you'll already know the power of their presence. If you don't have a pet, go and spend time with friend's animals or volunteer at an animal shelter. Offer to walk friends dogs or become part of an animal sitting network.

Some of my favourite days are when I get to look after my brother's cat, Crumpet. While she doesn't like to be picked up, she will spend time in your lap or nestled up to you in bed. Her presence is always a comfort and she seems to know when I'm coming to visit because she'll always leave me a gift on the doormat, whether it's a mouse or the wrapping from a greetings card. Well, it's the thought that counts!

Music plays an important part in our lives and is always there, whether it's in our car, on our phones, or playing in a store. We have so many memories connected to particular songs that we couldn't possibly count them all. Music can also be the perfect lift you need, even if it's only for the three or four minutes of a song. And it's never been easier to find, and connect, with that particular piece of music. If you don't know it, you can search for the lyrics that you do know and, before you know it, you're lost in a beautiful world of memories. Researchers are now discovering that each person has a unique balance beat, which is a sequence of notes that helps to pull a person back to a balanced state. If you find yourself listening to a particular song over and over, chances are that there's something in it that's making you feel great. Don't be ashamed of playing that song for all it's worth!

You can dictate your mood. Sometimes you may need a little help, but getting to a point where you feel happy and balanced doesn't have to be a struggle. Enjoy that journey of getting well again!

STRESS

Stress affects everyone whether it's through relationships, work, or general life. Knowing that it may be just around the corner can be just as painful as going through a period of stress. The swirling stomach, double vision, and clammy skin; we've all been there and it can affect us for days, weeks, and months.

Living with stress for any amount of time isn't healthy. It stops the body from resting and keeps you in a permanent state of fight or flight. Eventually stress becomes the body's default mode and we find it difficult to let go and relax.

Here's a newsflash; we're not supposed to be stressed, at least not for long periods of time. Stress is a reaction to a situation that we're not comfortable with. We may not know why we're stressed with the situation or it may be a reaction to something that has happened to us in the past. If it's a reaction to a past situation, take time to think about what may be triggering you and see if there are ways to work through the memories. Don't be afraid to get in touch with a therapist or counsellor if you need further support.

When stress hits, we may not be able to change the situation that's causing it, at least not straight away. There are many ways to help you relax and let go in the interim, many of which are talked about in this book.

People with mental health issues seem to suffer from stress far more than most and it can be the result of many different things. Imbalanced brain chemicals, life situations, the ongoing knowledge that there's something not quite right with you, lack of help or resources (be they medical, financial etc) can all play a part in how we feel. Eventually these situations become too much to bare and we fall ill, often setting our own recovery back by months or years.

The good news is that you're not alone. There are millions more like you, all feeling the strain and trying to work their way through it. The world isn't an easy place to live right now and there are many people and places that are popping up in order to help people through the hard times. As we've said before, if you need help don't be afraid to ask for it. Speak to your doctor and ask for for advice on where to get help; many have lists of government agencies and charities that will be able to help with your specific needs. Counselling and therapy services are often listed online or in doctors surgeries, libraries, and local phone directories. Mental health charities, many of which can be found listed in the same places as therapists and counsellors, will be able to offer support and advice.

While stress often feels like an all consuming cloud of darkness, there are many ways of combating and working through it. You don't have to spend your days dreading what the next moment will bring. You deserve to be happy.

HAVE NO FEAR

Fear is a mind-killer, a literal prison that we build around ourselves. Our worries come from everything around us; the media, friends, family, co-workers, people in the street, and overheard conversations. We're told that to step outside of this carefully crafted "normal" box is to commit a cardinal sin. To show that we're healthy, or sick, or somewhere in between is a crime.

It took me a long time to combat my own fears. When I first started writing I tried to control everything from where my name appeared to the reviews that were written. It was an exercise that took a lot of time and energy as well as causing a multitude of health problems.

Eventually I realised that the only world I could control was my own, so I began to shape it to my liking. I stopped reading my books reviews and started writing for myself. When I didn't feel like writing novels, I wrote short stories. When they lost their lustre, I turned to non-fiction.

I began treating people how I wanted to be treated. Love and respect were the order of the day and I chose to encourage rather than put down. Despite my minimum wage job, I stopped worrying about money and job security. I became of the mindset that there will always be something better around the corner.

There are still fears that haunt me but I'm slowly learning how to combat them. I try not to give in to the thought patterns that go around my head. One that always comes up is on New Year's Eve. I look back at the previous New Year's Eve and what I was doing on that night. Did a quiet night in cause me to have a bad year? Did a night out with lots of people cause me to have a good year? What do I have to do in order to avoid the pitfalls of the previous year?

What I've learned is that I need to follow my heart. If I want to go out and be with people, I'll do that. If I want to stay at home and have a quiet night, then that's what I'll do. What I'm doing on that night will not influence the next 365 days. What's in my head and how I deal with every day life will. What I need to be doing is improving myself in any way I can and not giving in to the fears that want to control my life.

Letting go of your fears can be terrifying. To stare them in the face and tell them that they no longer have any power of you takes great courage. But you can do it. You can start by listing them all. Take a piece of paper and write down everything that scares you. When you've finished, burn the paper and throw the ashes away. Confine your fears to the place that they belong; the trash. And then carry on with your beautiful life.

TALK ABOUT IT

One of the things I find difficult is talking about how I feel. When I'm on top of the world, I'll tell everyone who's willing to listen. But when I feel like giving up on life, I suddenly lose my voice and sink in to myself. It feels wrong to express my own pain when so many others in the world are suffering far more than I am. Even though all I want to do is cry, whenever someone asks me how I am, I always respond with, "I'm fine.".

Talking about how we feel isn't bad. We shouldn't feel as though we're adding to the world's suffering by expressing our own pain. We're not adding to the collective pain. By talking about how we feel, we're allowing ourselves to heal as well as using out stories to help others. As we've spoken about in "Stigma", there's still fear attached to mental health and every person who steps forward to speak of their own experiences is helping someone who may be too afraid to talk. By opening up about how you feel you may be giving courage to someone else to start their own process of healing.

We now live in a world that has more tools than ever to allow us to talk. Social media, blogs, forums, websites, Skype, FaceTime, email, text messaging... All of them, as well as physical face to face conversations, can be utilised to help you to talk about how you are feeling. Find a place that you feel safe; it may be with a therapist, a friend, or an online forum, and allow what's inside of you to come out. You don't even have to speak to another person. Keeping a journal or writing letters to yourself is just as useful and powerful as speaking to another human. Laugh, cry, shout, do whatever you need to in order to allow yourself to heal. The more you talk, the better you'll begin to feel. Before you know it, your pain will become happiness and you'll begin to spread your story to a world that needs it. You'll begin to help others who are still in the dark places that you have already walked through.

Don't be afraid to talk about what's going on inside of you. Don't keep it bottled up because mental health is a demon that can become a dragon, one that consumes you and drags you under. Allow yourself the space and the time to let all of your emotions come out. Once you're ready, you can step out and share your life with those around around. You can help to heal others and bring an end to the stigma that surrounds mental health. You are a valuable warrior, one whose voice is as powerful as any leader's.

Be proud of who you are and don't be afraid to speak up and make the world a better place.

CHOOSING A THERAPIST

Choosing a therapist doesn't have to be hard. Therapy may be covered by your insurance plan or be a part of your national health service. The best place to start is by speaking to your doctor. They may have a system in place where you're offered a set number of therapy sessions (which may later be extended if your therapist decides that it will be beneficial to you).

However, you can also contact therapists yourself because you need to find someone you're comfortable with. You may find contacts for practitioners at your doctor's surgery or online via Facebook or Google. Look at who is in your local area and see if any of them resonate with you. If they do, contact them (many offer the option of initially contacting them via email until you feel confident enough to speak either via the phone or face to face). Some may offer a free trial session to see if the two of you will be suitable to work together. They may also offer a free cancellation policy if you need to cancel a session.

Just as there are many different types of medicine, there are also different types of therapy. One may be more suitable for you than another or you may already know what kind of therapy you'd like to undertake. Investigate as many of the different therapies as you can. Types of therapy a therapist may practice include:

- Counselling

- Humanistic Therapies
- Cognitive Behavioural Therapy (CBT)
- Psychotherapy
- Behavioural activation
- Family or Relationship therapy
- Eye Movement Desensitisation and Reprocessing (EMDR)

Before you sign up with a therapist be sure to check their credentials. These should be listed on their website along with any governing bodies that they're a part of. They should also list their qualifications and whether they undertake regular training. Many will also "check in" with another therapist as part of their work. Be sure to ask questions before you sign up with a therapist. Your questions can include:

- Which therapy association or governing body are you a member of?
- Which types of therapy do you practice?
- Do you regularly update your training?
- Do you attend therapy sessions yourself or have another professional who you check in with?
- How much do you charge per session?
- Do I have to sign up for a set number of sessions?
- What happens if I have to cancel a session?
- Do you offer a phone or face to face consultation before I make a decision?

THE SOCIAL LIFE

Social media is a wonderful tool that allows us to keep in touch with far flung friends and family. We can stay in the loop with news, smile at our best friend's new baby, or chat the night away.

But social media, as many of us have discovered, can also be a dark place, one that fuels our fears and makes us feel insecure. There's always someone who is posting distasteful memes or talking politics that don't align with out own. We can wile away hours as we try and argue our case in the comments section of a triggering video. When everyone you know is on social media, it can be hard to log out.

There will always be people that you have to be friends with for the sake of keeping the peace but it doesn't mean that you have to see what they post. Unfollow anyone who makes you feel uncomfortable and report anyone who abuses or threatens you.

For several years I battled a drug addiction and now I find myself faced with a new, albeit digital, problem. I have an addictive personality meaning that I can find myself sucked in to the social media scene and not surface for days on end. Facebook runs whenever I'm on the computer, as does my email and website. I've turned off the notifications that appear on my desktop and I use a few programs to help limit my time on such sites. Leechblock, which runs on Firefox, allows you to block certain web addresses so you can still access your favourite sites without having to see certain people. StayFocused runs on Google Chrome and gives you a daily time limit to view your blocked websites before locking them (My time limit is set to a minute a day. A few days of accidentally going to blocked websites is enough to teach you not to go there!). It also has an option for completely cutting off internet access for a set amount of time.

There's plenty of programs and add ons on the market so find the ones that work best for you.

If you feel yourself being pulled in to the dark underbelly of social media step away and take time out. Remove the apps from your phone, or disconnect it from the internet altogether. Don't feel pressured to be online all the time. You may feel like you're missing out on something, but you're not. Real life is happening around you, right now, here in the moment. Real life doesn't happen on a computer screen. Take a walk. Sit by the window and watch the rain. Play with the cat. Read a book. Most of all, remember that you are more than your social media profile. You are more than your profile photograph, or your latest meal, or your current location. You are a living, breathing human being with emotions and a personality that can't be predicted or mimicked by a computer.

STAYING SANE AT CHRISTMAS...

...isn't easy.

I'm bipolar. It's something that I don't hide. Quite the contrary, in fact. I'm loud and proud about this unusual brain of mine, a condition which may, or may not, be the product of an overdose.

2016 was my first medication free Christmas. For over a decade, I took anti-psychotic medication to balance my brain in the wake of the overdose (I had come off my medication by Christmas 2015. But those drugs had been replaced by ones to combat sinusitis so this time last year I didn't know what planet I was on. It was actually quite nice!).

To say that December 2016 was stressful would be an understatement. I felt overwhelmed, tired, and sick. I could barely function but had to in order to get everything done. Three days before Christmas, I was on my hands and knees, sobbing with exhaustion and stress. I wasn't sleeping. I wasn't eating. I was vomiting from the tiredness. I was hallucinating. It was horrendous.

My apartment doesn't get decorated for Christmas. Not because I don't like Christmas but because the addition of lights and decorations overwhelm my already tired brain. Sure, I have a few ornaments that I put up. The cards that people give me decorate the lounge door so that I can see them every day. And I decorated the microphone stand that I use for interviews with a string of tinsel and small baubles (That might have to become permanent because it looks really cool!). But there's no tree, no music, and no glittering garlands.

Instead, I appreciate the decorations at other peoples houses, at work, and in the windows of shops. I *love* looking at photos of London's Christmas windows. But the abundance of bright lights, glittery decorations, and repeated Christmas music tires me out. The same goes for large gatherings. Anything over an hour spent in the company of a crowd of people makes my brain ache and my body weary (It's not you, honestly, it's not! Please don't take offence if I turn down an invitation. I really appreciate your love and company and would never not want to spend time with you.) And I realise that I need to have a space where I can escape from it all and get some rest.

Christmas can be a hard time for many people. There may be the feeling that they have to take part in everything that's happening. Saying no to an event or a party may be tough. They may feel that friends and family will frown on them if they decide that they need time out from the festivities.

On the flip side, they may despise Christmas and want nothing to do with it. Or have no one to celebrate it with (Thankfully, this year, there seemed to be many places that were hosting events for people who would be alone on Christmas Day. If you're alone next year, be sure to check local social media groups to see if there's anything happening).

Christmas shouldn't be a stressful time yet we seem to turn ourselves in to nervous wrecks for four weeks of the year. For some people, like myself, we pick up on the stress of those around us. When others are wound up, we get involved in those feelings, too, which only adds to what we're already feeling.

All of this can apply to any holiday, be it Christmas, Thanksgiving, Halloween, or any other time of the year when you may find yourself at social gatherings and other festive events.

Christmas, or any other holiday, doesn't have to be perfect. It shouldn't be all about whether everyone is included. Or how many gifts are under the tree. Or how many decorations we've put up. For many people, the chance to get together with others on one day of the year and celebrate is enough.

Wishing all of you a safe, prosperous, and healthy life!

SELF CONFIDENCE

Having confidence is a beautiful thing. With it, you feel as though you can change the world. Anything is possible and with confidence in yourself you can achieve whatever you set your mind to.

Often our mental health impairs our self confidence. Because of the way our brain functions, we can feel worthless and unable to make any kind of headway or find the success that our hearts crave. Because what's wrong with us is invisible we may feel that we're at the bottom of the list for a lot of things, be that help, promotions, or recognition. Often we may feel run down by the area we live in, have been bullied by others because of their perceptions of us, or because the world can be a dark place to live at times.

But there are many people with mental health issues who have fought adversity to become who they are today.

Ellen Degeneres (Talk show host and comedian) – Depression
Leonardo DiCaprio (Actor) – Obsessive Compulsive Disorder
J.K. Rowling (Author) – Depression
Carrie Fisher (Actress) – Bipolar Disorder (Type I)
Jim Carrey (Actor) – Depression
Elton John (Musician) – Bulimia
Gwyneth Paltrow (Actress) – Postnatal Depression

Catherine Zeta-Jones (Actress) – Bipolar Disorder (Type II)
Stephen Fry (Comedian, actor, writer) – Biopolar Disorder

You can do the same. Find that one thing that lights a spark in your heart and chase it for all you're worth. Use it to build up your confidence and to reach out in to the world.

For me, it was writing. This is my passion and my life. Whenever I have a free moment I'm either sitting here, at the computer, or scribbling away in a notebook. Writing gave me a voice that I didn't otherwise have and the internet gave me a place to use that voice. I had absolutely zero faith in myself when I started putting my work out there for the world to see. But, over time, the comments and emails began to roll in. Seeing that what I was writing was helping others, I found that my confidence grew. I was walking on air! So I wrote more and put that out there. My first novel won awards and I published three more books in quick succession. I kept on going until I found myself here, talking to you. And I feel honoured to be able to do this, to be able to share my journey with you. It means a lot to me that you've picked this up. Hopefully you're well on your way to healing yourself.

There are so many things that you can do to help build and boost your self confidence.

- Volunteer at places that inspire you whether that's an animal shelter or a hospital.

- Find classes at the local college or university that you want to take (Or take some online. Many universities now put their classes online for you to take for free).
- Join a gym or go to an exercise class.
- Offer to teach classes or help kids with their reading.
- Go to meet ups in your local area (Look at meetup.com to find some that suit you)

By following what you love, you can only build yourself up and help to make you, and the world, better.

THE PRISON IS A LIE

We're given labels from the moment we're born. Our gender, eye colour, and skin tone are all carefully noted. As we evolve, so more labels are added to our lives. These labels often come with negative connotations. We feel burdened by these titles, as if the words we're given to describe us are set in stone and unable to be changed. You may not be able to lose the extra weight but you need to know that you're not alone in the world.

These labels can drag us down, causing us to build walls round ourselves. We confine ourselves to the prison of being too fat, too thin, too tall, too short, using the labels as the bricks of the walls that surround us.

Mental health is awash with labels. Depression, Bipolar, Obsessive Compulsive Disorder... The list is endless. While the labels are given to us in a helpful manner, we can feel that our diagnosis is being used to define us as a person.

I could fill an entire book on the labels that have been attached to me. Short, fat, bipolar, female etc. You get the idea.

But those labels don't have to define you. They don't have to be a prison. They don't have to surround your mind with the grim, grey walls of what you've been told about yourself.

You have the key to open the prison door. Not your doctors. Not your family. Not your friends.

You.

You can open the door and decide to walk away from the words that have been attached to your physical being. You can say, "No more. I am not these words. I am not these labels. I am a human being with a soul and a spirit. I am far more than the words that have been bestowed upon me."

You may not grow taller or become thinner. But you can become you, the real you, the person who lives behind the height, weight, and diagnosis of your physical body. You can show the world that these labels can be crushed and that they have no meaning in this world.

You can destroy the prison that is within your mind. Only you can see if and only you can unlock the door. You are far, far more than the labels that have been attached to you.

Exercise

See yourself standing in a prison cell. The walls and ceiling are grey. Allow yourself to soak up the feelings of being trapped in the cell. You may feel loneliness, anger, despair, and anguish. Give yourself a moment to feel them.

Stretch your hands out in front of you and turn them palm upwards. See a large, golden key appear in your hands.

Walk to the cell door and insert the key in to the lock. Turn it and feel the door being to open.

Light streams in through the open door, chasing away the darkness and warming you. You step out of the cell and in to the light. Feel it wash over you and dissolve the negative emotions. Feel happiness, love, and acceptance fill your body.

You say, "I am free of the mental prison. Free to be myself. Free to love. Free to be me."

BODY

EVERYONE IS DIFFERENT

What makes you different to those around you? Is it your hair colour? Your eyes? Your voice? Your talents? Your experiences?

The media would like us to believe that everyone needs to look the same. Companies sell us products that are designed to play into our fears that we're not good enough. We're constantly told that we're too fat, too thin, too tall, too short. We feel small and inadequate and often go to great lengths so that we can fit in with what is seen as "Normal".

There is no normal. There are no standards that you have to live up to. Whatever you're being told to look like is an image designed by a company's design team and is than used to sell products and services to you.

Like everyone, I've tried to subscribe to the notion that there is a normal. I've tried to lose weight. I've tried to (unsuccessfully) wear make up. I've tried to keep with the ever-changing fashions. For me, it became too much and I loathed that I had to step up to some impossible standard in order to be accepted in the world. The whole experience tired and frustrated me until, one day, I said, "No more. I'm me. I'm not what the TV, magazines, and movies tell me that I should be". I didn't need acceptance that badly and so I laid down the idea that I had to be "normal" and went on my merry little way. Not everyone is going to fit in to whatever the media created standard is. In fact, only a tiny percent of the population will fit in to that standard, leaving the rest of us to buy the products, subscribe to the magazines, and pay for gym memberships in the vain hope that we, too, can achieve that goal.

Everyone is different. It doesn't matter who you are or where you live, you are different from the person who lives next door to you. Everything about you is as unique as a snowflake. You will look and sound different. The way you choose to dress may be different to those around you.

"Being normal" is mostly a herd mentality, one that we've carried with us through the generations. This mentality is what has protected us when we feel threatened. However, as life has moved on, this idea that everyone should conform to a set standard created by someone else is ludicrous. Our differences are what make us interesting. They're what pull us to other people. They're what allow us to find the people that become our tribe. They're what allow us to make differences in the world. Groove Armada put it perfectly in their song "If Everybody Looked The Same".

If everybody looked the same,
We'd get tired looking at each other.

Those words are so true at this time. We would get tired if everyone was the same. Being seen as different isn't a crime. Having differing opinions is what allows us to open up avenues to new ideas. Without differences there would be very little art. Without differences, we wouldn't have the technology that we have today.

You can choose how you look. You can choose what you do. You don't have to fit in to the constraints that society tries to impose on people. Don't be scared to be different. Don't be scared to stand out in the world. Don't be scared to be *you*.

WORK/LIFE BALANCE

Holding down a job when you have mental health issues can be tough. Truth be told, a lot of work environments can be hard if you have a disability. Bright lights, loud noises, strange people, and strict corporate environments can lead to more problems.

Going in to a place that isn't conducive to our well being can be difficult on a good day and unthinkable on a bad day. Trying to get people to understand that you may not always be one hundred percent can be like running a never-ending race. For a person with mental health issues, a job isn't just about the money. We may need something that feeds our soul and intellect. We may need to know that we won't lose our jobs because there are days when functioning isn't an option or we may need special adaptations to the environment.

I've worked my fair share of jobs over the years and nearly all of them have been a bad fit for me. From the loud pubs to the strict corporate environments, in a day and age when finding a job is a job in itself, it's hard to say "No" to any kind of offer. You never know if, and when, the next offer will appear so you have to take what's offered and hope for the best. These work places taught me something very valuable; that money isn't the most important issue. Your health is far more important than any pay cheque and if you feel ill, uncomfortable, or insecure at a job then you need to look for somewhere that will be more supportive of you.

Looking for something more suitable can be hard in an unstable economy and I'm not advocating that you quit your job right now. But there's nothing to say that you can't look at your other options. For me writing has been one of those options, along with my public speaking and editing work. I can expand on what I'm doing and make my portfolio bigger so that one day I can move on.

If jobs are limited in your area and you can't move to another area, try to switch off after work. Turn off your phone. Find a support group in your town or a forum online. Take a bath. Talk to a friend. Meditate. Listen to relaxing music. You can also use the light visualisations to protect and cleanse yourself.

Could you become self employed? Do you create anything that you could sell on Etsy, eBay and at craft fairs? Are you able to go and teach?

If moving is an option, think about what you'd like to do and see if there's any jobs that are a fit for you. Call companies that you're interested in. Even if they say no, you'd be surprised at how helpful they can be in putting you in touch with other potential employers. (One of my personal mottos is "You don't know until you ask". If you're scared of asking, work up the courage and do it. You'll honestly be surprised at what happens when you go in to something with the right mindset!)

You can do this, not because you have to, but because you're a person who deserves the best things that life has to offer!

ONE DAY AT A TIME

Every day can feel like climbing a mountain when your mental health isn't up to scratch. From the moment you wake up until the moment you drop back in to bed, life feels like it's out to grind you down. So it's no surprise that we often hide away inside of ourselves, scared to do anything that might upset our carefully balanced routine.

Looking at a new day is like looking at a blank notebook. There's so much possibility, so much that we could do. But then we start making notes of what we need, or want, to do and suddenly life feels like it's an uphill struggle. When you look at a year, the blank notebooks block out the chance of us seeing any happiness. We don't live. We survive. And that's incredibly sad.

Doing anything needs great mental and physical resources. It can take planning and preparation. So much effort to do even the tiniest chore eventually grinds you down until you... give up. You want to wither and fade, leaving no imprint of yourself on the world. Because why are you here and what's your purpose? Do we even have a reason for being alive?

One Day At A Time; that's the mantra here. Don't think about tomorrow. Don't think about yesterday. Just think about today. What needs to be done today? How can you accomplish it? More importantly, what would you *love* to do in order to allow yourself to be happy and healthy?

Life isn't about running from one chore to the next. The

dishes can wait, and so can the laundry. Dinner can be an hour earlier today. Or an hour later, depending on how you feel. The dust bunnies by the front door aren't going to mind waiting another day to be cleaned up.

Life is about living, feeling, and taking in the scenery. It's about experiencing great joys and crushing lows. It's about getting through the darkness and stepping in to the light. It's about appreciating the path you're on and knowing that there's a better place for you, a place that's beyond the stigma of your mental health. It's about learning how to be you without just being in survival mode.

Please don't just survive because there is so much more to this life. There's a beautiful world out there and it needs you to participate in its existence.

KEEP IT SIMPLE

One thing I've discovered is that the simpler my life is the happier I am. I don't do drama and I don't do clutter. I actively steer away from anything that could complicate my life because I can't think properly when I'm stressed and tired. In those times, my brain aches and I do little more than stare at the walls and worry about what may be. Someone causing problems for me? I cut them off. Apartment untidy? I clean it up and put everything away.

Disorder, whether physical or psychological, can cause problems for the brain and make you feel like you're out of control. It took me a long time to work out that, when my work space is a mess, I feel a mess. I can't concentrate and find it difficult to get things done. Having a space that's free of clutter can make you, and your brain, feel a lot better. Try and have somewhere clutter-free that you can go to when you need to rest. This space can be anywhere, even if it's only the corner of one room. Make it warm and homely and give it little touches that make it your own. Soft or coloured lights and gentle music or nature sounds can help your brain to relax. Spend time in this space whenever you feel like you need a break from the world.

I live by myself which makes keeping my space tidy a lot easier. Whenever I'm tired or whenever my brain is having a bad day, I curl up on the couch, pull my blanket around me and close my eyes. The room that I'm writing this book in has candles on many of the surfaces, plants on the desk and shelves lined with books. For me, it feels warm and happy and I enjoy the time that I get to spend in here (my desk isn't always tidy but I make the effort at least once a week to clear away any mess and wipe up the dust).

The same goes for other parts of your physical life, too. If you find yourself stressed at work and you notice that your desk is a mess, try tidying it. Add plants or other things that make you feel relaxed. Clear the receipts and old pieces of paper from your purse or wallet once a month. Shred the stack of old bills that you keep next to your desk. If you need to, invest in small cupboards to hide things away in. Buy a box file to put payslips and other essential paperwork in.

If you feel like your personal life needs organising and simplifying, buy a physical diary and wall calendar. I use the one on my phone but don't always see the reminders. Both the physical and phone diary as well as the wall calendar all have the same appointments listed in them so that I don't miss any (I still do from time to time but none of us are perfect!). To keep myself interested I have calendars made that show my favourite photographs. Then I have no reason not to look at them!

The same goes for the rest of your life and you'll find chapters within this book on how to keep your life as drama-free as possible. This isn't possible all of the time but there is a lot that you can do to keep it to a minimum.

CH-CH-CH-CH-CHANGES

David's Bowie's *Changes* is going through my mind as I write this chapter and the lyrics feel so poignant.

Turn and face the strain.

How many of us have had to do that? How many of us have felt the fear rise when we realise that our life is changing, even if we know those changes are for the better?

I know that I do. My mother tells me that I've always hated change. I get in to a comfortable little spot and then I don't want to move. She claims it's because I was born on a cold, snowy day and really didn't want to come out from the nice, warm womb.

And it's true. I'm not a big fan of change. Change makes me stressed and tired. Change makes me dig my heels in and resist everything that's coming. Change makes me want to hide under the bed and wait for it all to blow over.

But change happens whether we want it to or not. Friends come and go. Careers morph from one to another. Partners may flit through our lives. And each time, it feels like we're throwing a deck of cards in to the air and watching them fall.

We have to go through changes and there's nothing we can do to stop them. When we have mental health issues change often becomes more amplified. Because of the way our brains and bodies work we may have fallen in to a routine with medications, sleep patterns, and daily habits. We may have become used to waking at 7am and going to bed at 10pm. When 9pm rolls around, we know that it's time to take our medication while 5pm sees us eating dinner.

We panic when these routines are shaken up. Something as simple as arranging an evening out with friends can suddenly become a huge event. Will we be back in time to go to bed? Will we get the chance to eat at a regular time? We begin to feel paranoid and stressed as the event grows ever closer and may decide that, for our own peace of mind, cancelling will be better.

Change can be hard but it doesn't have to be impossible. I've learned that I need to talk about my fear of it, especially if it's a huge life changing event. As someone who prefers to work through things alone, talking about why I'm scared is tough. But it helps me to see that the change that's coming may not be all bad. Sure, it's going to hurt for a while. It's going to feel uncomfortable. But, at the end of the day, there may be something far better at the end of it.

Don't fear what's around the corner. And, if you do, take out the time to work out why you're scared. Once you've done that, smile, open your arms, and tell the world that you embrace all the change that's coming to you. Because you never know where it's going to lead you.

GETTING BACK TO NATURE

My body doesn't like exercise. Because I have a hormone imbalance I carry more weight than I should. And it doesn't matter how much exercise I do or how healthily I eat, that weight just won't shift.

But I love walking and exploring. I love seeing new things. On average, I walk between three and five miles a day and climb more stairs than I can count.

One of the pieces of advice that we've all been given is that doing some kind of movement, whether it's walking, running, dancing, cycling, climbing, or jumping up and down, is good for you. It can help to combat mental issues, gets you going, and lets you see the world around you.

And that advice is true. If I'm feeling fatigued, I'll make the short walk to the essential oil store just down the road (the store smells amazing, so it's a bonus pick-me-up!) or go to my brother's house to see his cat (and him, of course!).

Being outside also gives us a chance to top up on out vitamin D. Vitamin D is very good for helping with mental health issues and just fifteen minutes a day can help to make you feel better. If you live in an area that doesn't experience high levels of sunlight, especially during the winter months, you can invest in a sunlight lamp or visit a local health food store for vitamin D supplements.

When I'm in a new town or city I'll make a list of places

that I want to see and go exploring. Which is also good for honing photography skills or picking up inspiration for a new story.

If I'm in the countryside I'll amble along and take in the sights and sounds as well as soaking up the magic of not being surrounded by bricks and concrete.

Sometimes I'll just put my headphones on, find some music that I like, and walk. I'll go out with no specific purpose or destination other than the enjoyment of feeling my feet move against the pavement.

If you like being outside find a park or piece of countryside that you can be in. I know that this can be especially difficult if you live in a built up area so go looking for the nice parks and green spaces. If it's a beautiful day, take a picnic with you and find a spot to sit for a while.

If you like being with people, maybe find an exercise class to take part in. I know that this can be tough but maybe start with the easier classes where not everyone will be a pro (things like Zumba Gold are good for this) and work your way up.

Maybe join a gym or get workout DVDs. There's also a lot of workout videos on You Tube now and there are online communities where you can get encouragement and support from around the world.

Or maybe crank up your favourite song, sit in your favourite chair, lift your feet and wiggle your toes.

Movement, no matter how much or how little you do, is good for the soul. You'll feel so much better for being able to open your body up and prepare it for the life that you're supposed to lead. It doesn't matter how much you do, moving your body is a great way to remind you that you're alive.

So plug your headphones in, find your jam, and do a little wiggling!

PUSHING THROUGH THE PAIN

The voice in your head that says you can't do this is a liar.

My immune system is broken. I make no bones about it, nor how it came to be that way. This is what nearly 15 years of illegal, and prescription, drug use does to you. It might not happen to everyone but, for me, it's left me having to take life at a slow, steady pace. With love and care my body will hopefully repair itself. For the time being, I'm eating a healthy diet and loading up on vitamins and minerals. And I'm lucky to be alive, something that I'm eternally grateful for.

With it comes a whole slew of side effects. The exhaustion is crippling and some days it starts before I've even stepped out of bed. My energy levels go up and down more often than a roller coaster. And my social life is non-existent because I'm either too tired, am recovering from some virus, or am trying to avoid another. It's not you, it really is me!

But all of this has given me the time to follow my heart. It's given me the chance to search deep inside of myself and rediscover those hopes and dreams that I'd previously thrown to the wind. It's allowed me to sit back and start working on these things at a slower pace. Things may seem like they're not happening but, deep down, you know that there's a shift happening and that there is something bigger just over the horizon.

Your dreams don't happen overnight. They take a lot of work. So what happens when the inevitable tiredness raises its ugly head? How do you push through the pain and weariness to keep on going?

Often this is when people stumble and stop. The exhaustion and the effort force them to stop and make do with the life they have. Their mind tells them that everything they're working for doesn't exist and that there is no use in carrying on. Why bother when there will be nothing to show for it at the end?

But, rather than going wrong, what if it all goes so right? What if everything you've ever wanted is just going to take one more little push?

When the doubt and the exhaustion arrive stop for a few days. Take a step back and enjoy the life that you have right now. Look at where you are and all that you've accomplished. Those amazing photographs that everyone comments on? Yep, you took those. That story that everyone is raving about? Yep, you wrote that. That piece of art that's hanging in the little coffee shop in town? Yep, you created that. The song that a stranger is currently passing around social media? Yep, that's yours.

When I'm too tired to move I stop and step away from my computer. I go and lie on the sofa. Or read a book. Or listen to some music. When the doubt appears, I think back on the wonderful reviews and comments I've had about my writing. It's the push I need to pick myself up the next day and do a little more.

Just because the big things haven't arrived yet doesn't mean that they won't. They will but you have to keep pushing on through to reach them. Enjoy what you have right now and, once you feel ready, go back to what you were doing.

You can do this, one step at a time...

THE POWER OF PLAY

We're told that, once we reach a certain age, we must leave our childhood behind. No longer should we run through the snow or laugh at cartoons. Our favourite books and toys must be put away or given to other people. When these objects leave our lives, a little part of us goes with them.

However, in recent years reliving your childhood has become big business. There's adult colouring books and giant ball pools. Uber delivers puppies and kittens to offices. Foods that we'd forgotten about suddenly make a comeback. Embracing the child within you has never been so easy or so cool.

And that's because play is good for you. Just as when you were a child, play helps to stimulate you and keep you active. The rewards of letting go and losing yourself in the latest colouring book or Disney film can be incredible for your brain, allowing serotonin, the happy chemical, to flow .

Play helps to relax you and gives you the opportunity to laugh, feel rested, and to reconnect with the world around you. Work places are embracing the power of allowing employees to build Lego models. Stores are once more overflowing with our favourite childhood toys (I have a Foo Fighters themed Matchbox car that I idly push around my desk while I'm thinking). Cinemas are filled with the movie versions of our favourite comic books. Play allows serotonin – the happy hormone – to flow through our systems and make us feel, well, happy.

No longer are we restricted to what we believe we're supposed to do as adults. We're not here to sit at a desk for forty hours a week and spend our weekends cleaning the house and doing the laundry. We're not here merely to work and die. We're not here just to exist. We're spiritual beings whose hearts and souls need to be nurtured just as much as our bank balances do. As you give yourself more freedom so the rest of your life will fall in to place. You don't have to lead a regimented life thinking that you have to live the get up-work-come home-eat-sleep routine. Do you notice how stressed you feel when you do that? That's not what we're supposed to do and yet we do because we believe it's what leading an adult life is about.

We're allowed to run in the snow, climb trees, build pillow forts and doddle interesting images. We can lose ourselves in the latest young adult novel or buy tickets to the latest Pixar movie.

You have permission to allow yourself to be that child. Explore. Laugh. Love. Live. And see the world through innocent eyes.

THE LONELIEST ROAD

There are some periods in our life when we find ourselves alone. We may still be surrounded by family and friends but these people may not understand the journey you're taking. The path you're walking may be one relating to your career, relationships, or another aspect of your life. You may not want others to know what you're working through or they may have asked you not to speak about it. It's a hard choice between living a life that seems normal and following what's going on in your heart.

Taking a life journey by yourself can be daunting. You're alone with no one to talk it and your only company is yourself. It's not a straight road and is one that is often fraught with sharp turns and shadowy embankments. You don't know what you're going to find around the next corner and your drive to find out won't allow you to stop.

But the loneliness can become crippling. Everyone needs someone to talk to and to find reassurance for their actions. The longest, loneliest road often doesn't have these people and the person taking this journey can find themselves isolated and depressed. They want to talk. They want to share what they've seen and what they've found. Yet, all too often, the understanding souls they can talk to just aren't there.

The creative arts are like this and I've known many people who've stood on this road and asked themselves what they're doing. They've debated turning back and giving up because they can't abide the darkness that consumes them. They hate being alone and want someone to share the joy of the journey with.

I'm going through this at the moment. While I watch my friends and family prepare for huge, life changing events I find myself sitting here with piles of paperwork as I try and get my latest project off the ground. There's no promise that it will work but I can't sit back and think "what if?". I'm driven to do it and only I can put in the work that will make it come to life. The risk and the not knowing is part of this journey that so many people take. Yet, along the way, I can't help but feel the pangs of loneliness as I watch people I know gather, laugh and celebrate.

Yet I've also seen so many people who've reached the end of the road and found amazing things at the end. Much like the proverbial pot at the end of the rainbow, they've hit the jackpot in more ways than they can imagine.

The journey may be long and it may be hard. It may seem to be fraught with danger and darkness. But good things can only come from it. Never give up and know that you're never alone.

ALONE TIME

The issues that we face can make us feel isolated, our brains making us feel as though no one else will understand us. Even though millions of other people may have similar issues to our own, they affect each person very differently and make explaining what's happening difficult.

Sometimes, though, we need the alone time to rest and figure out who we are. We may have issues that we need to work through or just want some time off from the world.

Being alone is not a bad thing. It takes great strength to spend days, weeks, months, or years by oneself. Strength that we may believe that we've forgotten. You're not weak, not in the slightest. You spend every day battling something that no one else can see.

Like many people who've had something go wrong with their brain, I find my alone time to be rewarding. It's my way of escaping from the noise of the outside world. I don't have to listen to depressing news, or pick up painful emotions from other people. In this little cocoon I rest and reset myself, ready for whatever the next day brings. Here I can listen to music, meditate, read, and write. I can explore worlds that others may not see, completely undisturbed by the one outside.

There are times when I crave human company and, in those moments, I go and visit family or friends. I'll walk to the local supermarket, go to a concert, or spend time in the nearby coffee shop. Being alone doesn't have to be a time of deep depression. Instead, it can be a time of liberation and learning to be comfortable in your own skin.

I needed to learn to be comfortable with myself. While I was at university, I hopped from one relationship to another, determined to find "The One". I was scared of being alone but, in my hunt, I found that there was loneliness even in the most loving of relationships. I didn't find "The One" and I learned that, for a while, I needed to be by myself, at least for the time being.

It took me a long time to feel comfortable with myself and to learn to enjoy my own company. For the first few years, I hopped from one hobby to another as I searched for another human love. That love never came. Instead, something else happened.

I found myself falling in love with myself. Through this adventure I learned to love all the little quirks that make me, well... me.

You don't have to fall in love with yourself during your time alone. Maybe you'll fall in love with the stars. Or the moon. Or that book you bought four years ago and haven't yet read. Being alone isn't a crime for having an illness, nor is it necessary. But you may find that a little time away from the world, whether it's five minutes or five months, helps to relieve whatever your brain decides to throw at you.

LOVE YOURSELF

Loving yourself are words that we don't hear very often and it's a concept that can be hard. How do we love ourselves when our health makes us feel so low?

Giving yourself the attention and space that you need can be difficult. We spend our lives running from homes to jobs to medical appointments to schools. We may find that we spend more time looking after others than we do ourselves. Living with mental health issues often makes us more inclined to reach out and help others, our own understanding of what's happening able to ease another person's pain or discomfort.

But, at some point along the road, we stop. We can't go on, the stress and exhaustion of trying to please and look after so many people having taken over. Our bodies begin to wear out and our mental health suffers even more.

I've lost count of how often I've done this. More than I'd like to hazard a guess at. And each and every time, I've ended up in bed, crying to myself because I can't sleep. My brain will ache and my body will be exhausted. But still I won't be able to sleep as a million and one different thoughts whirl around my head.

We have to love ourselves. We *need* to love ourselves. Giving ourselves space and time is important. I know people who don't reply to emails, messages, or their phones on a weekend. I limit some of the events that I get involved with as well as only sporadically checking my email.

It took me a long time to realise that I gave a lot of myself to others without really doing anything for myself. My stress levels were off the charts. I wasn't sleeping, and eating was just something I did to keep myself going. So I'd step away and recharge myself before doing it all over again.

Eventually, even that became too much and I realised that I had to step away either for a longer period or permanently. I gave up the writing website I ran. I stopped keeping my phone close by. I began ignoring my email. I refused to reply to people straight away.

It was the first step to looking after and loving myself. While I still reach out and help people, I'm more likely to look at myself first before I get involved. How am I feeling? Am I stressed? Tired? Hungry? Run down? Will I be able to cope with someone else's problems, possibly for the long term?

If the answer is no to any of those questions, I politely decline and step away.

But loving yourself isn't all about giving yourself space. It's about doing the things that you enjoy. These days I read more of the books that I want to read rather than what I think I should be reading. I take long baths. I cook nice foods. I make myself feel good. Because feeling good about yourself puts you in the best place possible to help heal yourself and those around you.

LISTEN TO YOUR BODY

We live in a world that wants us to be doing something twenty four hours a day. We're constantly connected to each other, only a phone call, text message, or email away from family, friends, and work colleagues. The news is forever being shown to us, our worlds filled with disasters, pain, and death. We're encouraged to never turn off, never disengage, never take our eye off the ball that is our ever changing world.

But we're human. We grow tired and weary. We get sick. There are times when all we want to do is climb in to bed and sleep.

Do it. Don't listen to what the people around you say. If they're saying you need to work an eighteen hour day, ignore them. Kick off your shoes, drop on to the couch, and relax. Because, at some point, your body will get whatever it's demanding of you.

I've been one of those people. I still am to some degree. I've burned the midnight oil. I've worked until I can't see straight. I've kept going until I'm vomiting from exhaustion. And I've done it because the people around me – family, friends, people on social media, the news – have told me that I have to do it. Because, in this world, that's what's expected of you; to work until you drop.

Sickness hasn't been a stranger thanks to pushing myself so hard. I've had several breakdowns and each and every time I've put on a smile and worked on through it. Because that was what was expected of me.

Everyone else was doing the same thing so why shouldn't I? Everyone else was pushing themselves to the brink of exhaustion, so why shouldn't I? Everyone else was tired, tense, and broken from the stress they'd bought on themselves, so why shouldn't I? Doing so would apparently make myself, and the world, better. And if I didn't do it, if I didn't comply to these worldly standards, then I'd be seen as weak and lazy.

Instead, I found myself going round in circles, stuck in jobs that depressed me and working on projects that didn't inspire me. I'd push myself to the limit, become ill, and, once I was well enough, start the cycle again. My body was lashing out at me time and again, warning me that, sooner or later, I'd end up in a place where I could no longer look after myself. Finally, and with help from several friends, I realised what I was doing and became determined to stop it.

I trimmed my life down. Gone were the multitudes of projects that everyone else wanted me to work on. I began to focus on the things that I wanted to be involved with. I got rid of the physical clutter and I turned my apartment in to a little sanctuary of peace and calm. I began turning my phone off and installed blocking programs on my computer so that I couldn't spend hours surfing social media.

Most of all, I stopped listening to the people around me and began listening to my body. When it said sleep, I went and slept. When I wanted to eat, I ate. I wrote when it wanted to write and read when it wanted to read.

There's a lot of noise around us, noise that comes from so many different sources, making it difficult to listen to ourselves. Take time to stop and truly listen to what your physical being is saying.

LIVE HEALTHY

A key part of living with mental health issues is to lead a healthy life. This doesn't have to be complicated nor does it have to be expensive.

I know that when you have mental health issues living on easy to prepare meals can literally be a lifesaver, especially if you've had a tough day. But eating well is a good place to start when it comes to your mental health. Starchy carbohydrates such as white bread and pasta can make us feel more tired than we already are. Replacing them with whole-wheat bread and pasta is a good start.

I'm a huge fan of stir fry and I've found that egg noodles tend to make me feel bloated and lethargic. When I switched to rice noodles, the problem went away.

Eat as much fruit and as many vegetables as you can. Living well doesn't mean you have to give up your favourite foods. It just means adding in more natural foods. If you feel like you're lacking in certain vitamins and minerals, visit your doctor and see if they can recommend supplements. Often the staff at health food shops are also trained to give advice on vitamins and minerals.

Exercise is something else to consider. The chapter "Getting Back to Nature" talks about the benefits of being outside. However a short walk, whether it's around your block or just to the store, is a great way to kick start your body's healing process. You may find yourself drawn to a gym, exercise class, or some other form of exercise. But it's true that exercise definitely helps the body when it comes to working with your mental health. Being outside, even for as little as ten minutes, can help you get your recommended daily dose of Vitamin D. Vitamin D is extremely useful when it comes to living with mental health issues as it helps you to feel more upbeat. And, let's face it, there's nothing better than sitting in a park on a sunny day, right?!

Getting enough sleep is another important factor in keeping yourself healthy. Admittedly this can be extremely difficult when your brain is chattering away to you. There are nights when I don't sleep at all, tossing and turning as I watch the clock's hands slip through the wee hours, until finally I have to get up and go to work. I've given myself a regular bedtime of 10pm and normally wake up at about 5 or 6am. I've found that having things like a Himalayan salt lamp and lavender oil in the bedroom help me to relax and fall asleep. Another recommendation is to not have mobile phones and tablet computers in the room with you and to stop using them thirty minutes before you go to bed. That can be hard, especially if you're waiting for important updates. But I've found that it helps to leave my phone elsewhere in the apartment after doing a very crude experiment. One night I decided to see what would happen if I slept with my phone beside my bed. I used it just a few moments before I turned my light out and had one of the worst nights sleep that I'd ever had. So the phone now stays outside of the bedroom. Sleep is important as it helps the brain to sort through all its information as well as get the rest it needs. Like your body, it's also a working a organ and needs time to shut off and reset.

Having a healthy life really can make all the difference. Make the most of the life you've got!

YOU ARE NOT YOUR BODY

Well, you are because you have to live in it. But you're far more than the flesh and bones that make up your exterior. You're a spiritual being having a very human experience.

Mental health can play havoc with our exterior as well as our interior. What's happening on the inside, even in our brain, can manifest through our physical form. Medications, for example, can become a minefield when you're trying to look after yourself. Some may make you lose weight while others will pile on the pounds without you even trying.

I've been at both ends of the spectrum. I've taken medications that have made me lose weight. At the other end of the scale, I've taken ones that have made me put on weight whenever I've so much as looked at food. Weight that I'm still battling to lose.

But that's not all that there is to us. You a person with hopes and dreams, fears and anxieties. Everyone is different, their personalities, looks, and the path they're walking in this life making them as individual as snowflakes. You are worth far more than what your body looks like.

Unfortunately we live in a world that does judge us by our appearances. We can be too tall, too short, too thin, too fat, too much, or too little of anything. Words that are said to us can be cripplingly, more so when we're mentally fragile. Getting beyond those words and to a place of peace can be a battle in itself.

But know that you're not alone. Know that you are not the only person who is going through this. Whenever someone throws harmful words in your direction, ask why they're doing it. What makes them feel insecure enough that they have to lash out at another because of that person's appearance? Why can't they see past the exterior and to the beautiful person that lies beneath the skin? Chances are that the person who is saying such things won't admit up to any wrongdoing. But know that, deep down, they're hurting probably far more than you are. For them, the work to get to a place where they are comfortable is like climbing a mountain.

It's taken me a long time to see past the exterior of my person and see the inside. See the real me. See all that I can be. See that I'm far, far more than what the outside of my body says that I am.

You are *not* what other people say you are. You are *not* what the bathroom scales say you are. You are *not* what your head is telling you that are. You are *not* what the mirror says that you are.

You are far more than what your body. *You* are beautiful. *You* are talented. *You* are living the way that you want to live. *You* are wanted. *You* are loved. *You* are needed. *You* are perfect just the way you are.

HAVE A LIFE CLEAR OUT

Do you ever feel overwhelmed by the amount of stuff that you have? That stuff could be physical items, friendships, or relationships. There are days when you take a look at your life and think "How the heck did I wind up with all of this?".

Stuff, no matter what it is, can be overwhelming. Just taking a look at my bookshelves gives me anxiety. There's so many books and little bits and pieces that sometimes I don't know what I'm going to do if I move again. Where will I store my books? What will happen to all the pieces that people have sent me? There are some days when I want to clear them all out and start afresh.

To some degree, I have done. Every time I move I sort out everything that I can bear to part with. Everything gets boxed up and goes to the charity shop or to friends who can make better use of it than I can.

Having a clear space can be good for your brain. Space allows your brain to rest and reset itself. My bedroom, for example, is the space that has the least clutter. Bar my bed, a wardrobe, two small chests of drawers, and two pieces of artwork, there's nothing. The walls have been left in their original white and there's a blackout blind over the window. I wanted it to resemble a hotel room as much as possible, somewhere that I'd be happy to fall in to after a long day.

And it works. Having very few items in the room with me allows my brain to switch itself off far quicker. I rest easier and feel far more refreshed.

Take a look around where you live. If you feel overwhelmed by how much you have, take a look at what you could donate, sell, or give away. The rule that I live by is that if an item hasn't been used or worn for a year, then it's given away to someone who will make better use of it.

You can do the same with friendships. We all have those friendships that we want to release, the people who we feel weigh us down. You may feel as though you can't talk to the person about how the friendship makes you feel. Or, if you do, you may find that neither of you can reach a satisfactory conclusion.

Take a look at how that person impacts your life and how they make you feel and slowly start to pull away. This may be painful but know that the pain will pass. Sometimes it is for our own good to allow others to leave our lives. Never try to hold on to a friendship that is primarily negative as it isn't good for either of you.

You, and your brain, deserve to rest. Make the most of the space you have and make it beautiful for you!

THE HEARTBEAT OF OUR LIFE

"I don't believe in guilty pleasures. I think you should like what you like." — Dave Grohl (Reddit AMA)

Music is a far more powerful tool than we give it credit for. Put your hand on your chest. Feel that? That's your heart *beating*. Music lives within all of us right from the moment we're conceived. It's something that you live with right from the very first seconds of life. Music has the ability to heal, something that the Chinese have understood for many years. Their character for"Music" is incorporated into the one that means "Medicine". The Chinese character for music also has a second meaning: delight and happiness. Music is being used the world over to help unlock the minds of dementia patients. Every human being has a "balance note", a harmonic that they respond to and that helps to keep the body and mind healthy. When they feel happy, they listen to a lot of music with this frequency (which may explain why you listen to a song on repeat). When they feel sad, or ill, they'll search through their music until they find that frequency to help rebalance themselves. Many people, myself included, use music to help us get through tough times. Again, many of us can trace passages in our life through certain songs. Music is everywhere within ourselves and nature. NASA have shown that even the universe sings to us.

When it comes to mental health, music can be as

important as any kind of medication or therapy. Why? Because it makes us feel *good*. Music, like many other things, can release the feel good hormones in to our system. Music can be used to help battle the pain, depression, and loneliness that we feel. Music can help us to feel connected in a world that wants us to feel disconnected from one another.

We are more than our physical bodies. We are more than just skin and bones. We have fire and drive living deep inside of us, a spirit that nothing can quash. If someone knocks us down, we lick our wounds and get back up.

Just like music, we vibrate with an unseen energy. We *are* energy. Every little part of us is. We're constantly putting it out in to the world and it returns to us from the people around us.

We're constantly finding songs and sounds that resonate with us and that speak to that unquenchable spirit that lives within us. Each song is a moment in time, a piece that holds far more memories than any photograph ever will. Songs relate to places we've been, people we've met, and experiences we've had. Our back catalogue of music is as big as any that's out there. And each of our personal playlists, the ones we've created throughout our lives, are as different as we are to one another.

Play your favourite songs. Relive the memories. Allow yourself to let go and feel good, lost in the sound of someone else's creation. Sing. Dance. Laugh. Cry. Cling to the good moments. And let the old ones be taken by the wind. Don't be ashamed of who you are and never be ashamed of your personal playlist.

SPIRIT

YOU ARE AMAZING

Never forget...

You are beautiful, both inside and out. Don't let the media, or anyone else, tell you that you're not.

You are talented. Just because you aren't where you want to be yet doesn't mean that you won't get there.

You are loved. Your family and friends love you as much, if not more, than any partner may do.

You are kind. Don't allow your confidence to be broken by others perceptions of you. Their actions speak more of them than they do of you.

You are desirable. Someone may not be knocking at your door right now but you don't know who will appear tomorrow.

You are courageous. You may be waking up to a world that wants to bring you down. Yet every day you face it with courage and dignity. That takes more strength than you can possibly imagine.

You are not a failure. So you're angry/hurt/sad? This will pass. It's what you allow it to do to you that matters. Don't dwell on it; you're human and have emotions. But move on from it.

You are an inspiration. People will look up to you for many reasons but they may never tell you. Praise the people who inspire you.

You make the world a better place just by being in it. Keep loving and living because your life, and your spirit, are needed.

You are amazing. Never forget that.

BE TRUE TO YOURSELF

When your brain doesn't work properly it can be very difficult to know who you are. You may have been told by doctors, therapists, and well meaning people that you need to look, act, or speak a certain way. Or you may feel like you have to put on a front for the world or hide behind a completely different identity. Yet your heart and soul may be telling you something completely different.

We all have that personality that we show the world. More often than not, when you're not feeling well, your personality will be one that tells the people around you that you're doing great. You may smile when you feel like crying. Or get dressed up when you want to be in bed.

Like many people, I've been there and done that. I've had the Rachael that only people outside of my home have seen. I've dressed how people think I should dress. I've listened to people and tried to be the person that *they* believe I should be.

And it was one of the hardest things I've ever done. Trying to keep that facade up was time consuming and draining. Being fake Rachael made me depressed because I thought that I had to look like the women in the magazines. I thought that fake Rachael had to be skinny, wear dresses, and generally be a girly-girl. I was dying inside.

In the end, I gave up. I was determined to love my

short, curvy body and collection of physical imperfections. I would revel in my geekiness and celebrate my differences. I would love everything that made me utterly unique. The dresses were replaced with jeans and a wardrobe of band t-shirts. Make up was only worn on special occasions. The dull home furnishings were replaced with concert posters and an ever growing collection of music memorabilia. I was determined to be the real me and it feels amazing.

As I changed so did the people around me and old friends were replaced by ones who were more aligned to me. They're people who wanted an authentic life experience and who weren't scared of being who they're truly supposed to be.

To show the world who you truly are is a terrifying prospect. You may feel fragile or believe that you're too broken to be true to yourself. But only you know what lies in your soul. Only you know the person you're supposed to be. Only you know what your life path looks like. Only you can make the changes to become the person that longs to escape from deep inside of you. Only you can find the courage to take that first step out on to a brand new path.

If you step outs of your shell, you'll realised that there's a beautiful new life that awaits you, one where you'll be happier than you've ever been. You can find your amazing self.

EASY TARGET

Having mental health issues means that, at times, you can find yourself in groups of people very much like yourself. You find comfort and solace with people who are going through the same thing that you are. You're vulnerable, something that we're encouraged to be if we're taking medication that numbs the emotions. We're told that to feel and be open about these feelings is good. So when people come along and show an interest in us we may find ourselves revealing more than we wish to give away.

If you're not careful this information can be used against you, to grind you down and make you feel even more worthless. I was in just such a friendship. Someone spotted that, post-coming off my medication, I was in a weak place. I was figuring out myself, and the world, and they used that to their advantage. By saying that they understood what I was through, they won my trust and soon had all the information they needed to turn my world upside down.

Before I knew what was happening this person was using psychological tactics to turn me against my family and friends. They made me question my whole existence and whether my carefully planned withdrawal from medication was a good thing. I was told to correct problems that only this person could see. When I thought that I'd mended myself they found another non-existent problem to berate me for.

After nine months, the only escape I could see was to end my own life. This person, someone I'd labelled as a friend, had pushed me in to one of the deepest, darkest depressions I can remember. They had a hold on me and were a weight around my neck that I couldn't release myself from. When they sensed that I was beginning to pull away, they threatened to end my writing career or expose me in some other way. The threat was enough to make me stay, leaving in fear at what this person's next move may be.

Thankfully modern technology has made it easy to rid ourselves of such people. Phones now block numbers without you having to call your provider. Social media allows us to do the same, not questioning us when we reach for the block or report buttons. The police are now far more understanding if you need assistance in ridding yourself of unwanted attention.

After my encounter with this person, it took a long time for me to rebuild my confidence and self esteem. There are still days when I doubt myself. But I'm in a far better place than I was all those months ago.

Don't let anyone take your power away from you. If a person you meet doesn't feel right to you then you are under no obligation to let them in to your lie. Learn to say "No" to friend requests and invitations. It can be hard at first but, in the long run you'll so much better for it. The world needs you to be a beautiful, happy, and healthy person.

NOT MY CIRCUS, NOT MY MONKEYS

I love that saying! Every time I see it, it makes me laugh. Translated from Polish, *Not my circus, not my monkeys* basically means "Not my problem".

You can experience a lot of drama and nonsense when you have mental health issues. Things may arise among friends, during group therapy sessions, in the work place, or in any number of other locations or situations. You may find yourself caught in the crossfire of drama that's been spawned on a website. I use the word "drama" to describe any kind of chaos, stress, or pain that's brought in to your life by someone, or something, else.

Many of us know what it's like to struggle in life. We may have experienced poverty, homelessness, loneliness, or any number of other issues. Because of this we have the experience to help people who are going through something similar.

I seem to attract people who aren't always honest in their dealings with others. They may set out to use me for their own ends, or to borrow substantial amounts of money. Often, such people bring drama and heartache with them and threaten my own well being. Because of some of the things that I've been through in my own life, I welcome them in, believing that I can help them. Unfortunately, their intentions aren't always in alignment with my own. It took me several years, and a lot of drama, before I learned to recognise those kinds of people. I now put the brakes on those friendships before they have a chance to flourish. It may seem harsh but I'd rather focus my attention on people whose intentions are the same as my own.

Learning the phrase *Not my circus, not my monkeys* was a light-hearted and humorous way of dealing with the issues and drama that came in to my life. It allows me to take a step back and look at the situation more deeply, often making me realise that the problems that are coming in to my life aren't of my creating. None of us should have to deal with the other peoples drama but we do because our hearts are big and our spirit is kind.

Big hearts and kind spirits are what this world needs. But they also get damaged very easily, often making us cynical and disillusioned. When we've been hurt, whether it's once, twice, or a hundred times, we don't want to reach out and help others who may need us. But we're here for a reason, just as there's a reason behind the experiences that we've had. We're here to help one another and to reach in to the darkness and pull others out. But we can't do that if we constantly find ourselves wrapped up in the drama that's laid on our doorstep.

You know what the drama feels like. We all know those sleepless nights and strained days that it cane bring. Every time you feel yourself getting pulled in to someone's nonsense, take a step away, draw in a deep breath, and repeat these words: Not my circus, not my monkeys.

POSITIVE AFFIRMATIONS

In the chapter "Mental Aerobics" we talked about how words have power and that changing a single word in sentence can make a big difference in how you feel and how your perceive yourself. Say them to yourself until you start to feel better, and then keep on going. You can use these words whenever, and wherever, you feel the need to. There's no designated time or place that you should use them. Even if you're not feeling down, take a look at them and remind yourself that you're a beautiful soul.

I am loved.

I am wanted.

I am needed.

I am worthy.

I am beautiful.

I am strong.

I am protected.

I am happy.

I am peaceful.

I am unique.

I am deserving.

I am light.

I am successful.

I am in control.

I am not broken.

I am rested.

I am more than good enough.

I believe in myself.

I can do whatever I put my mind to.

My life is not a bad life.

Tomorrow is another day and another chance to start afresh.

This is my life and no one can take it from me.

No one has the right to exert their power over me.

WHEN THE DARKNESS FALLS

My entire body, from my head to my feet, aches. I've been to work and now I'm in bed before the last rays of the sun have touched the horizon.

When my depression kicks in I go from enjoying life to sitting on my couch, eating popcorn, and binge watching shows on Netflix. For someone who ordinarily doesn't watch a lot of TV I sure can watch a lot when the mood suits me. Instead of wanting to live and create and laugh I begin to live minute to minute, counting them down until I can go to bed or make another bowl of popcorn. I begin to worry about *everything* and, in the morning, I climb out of bed, plaster on my best "I'm okay" face, and go to work.

I don't like living with the darkness. Personally, I don't know anyone who likes having depression. I know a lot of people who want to get away from it and that partly what this book is about. It's about giving you the tools that I've used so that you can live a happy, healthy, and purposeful life.

When I came off of my medication I knew that I had two choices. I could dwell in the darkness and spend the rest of my life wondering what may have been. Or I could walk in to the light and live a better life. I could become a better person, one who wasn't so bitter, jealous, and angry (Trust me, those emotions still rear their heads at times, just like every other emotion. But it's choosing not to give them space in your head that counts). I could love those around me and hopefully, in the process, encourage them to become the best person that they can be.

Making the decision to leave the depression behind is one of the best you'll ever make. And making that decision is the first step in successfully leaving the darkness behind you. Sure, it'll come and visit from time to time and the fight can be long and painful. But you'll be strong enough to do battle with it.

Looking after yourself is the best thing that you can do. Make yourself do the things that you don't want to do (going to work, doing the shopping, making that phone call etc) but also make sure that you do some of the things that you love.

Sit on the couch. Eat the popcorn. Watch the TV show. Sing your heart out. Write a poem. Dance in the rain. Don't beat yourself up too much and be kind to yourself. And know that tomorrow the sun will rise and a new day will begin.

You can win. You just have to make the decision to step out of the darkness and in to the light.

YOU'RE NOT HERE JUST TO EXIST

You're not here just to exist. You're not here just to go through the daily grind and fall in to bed. You're not here just to be a statistic, or a name, or a number on a form.

You're not a human doing.

You're a spiritual being having a human existence.

How many of us have, at some point in our lives, sat there and said, "What am I here for? Everything feels pointless. I feel like I just... exist."?

Probably most of us. And it's no wonder that we say and think such things.

Over the years, I've met many people who have unique and incredible talents. Yet, because of their circumstances, they decide that a life of monotony is all that they deserve. I've met the photographer who could make the most boring landscape look beautiful but who decided that his talents weren't little more than a hobby. I've met the musician who decided that being a driver for a ride-share company was better than taking the risk to try and make it in the music industry. I've met the writer who decided to stick at a desk job rather than try and pursue their wonderful ideas. Each and every person has broken my heart as I watch their talents slowly go to waste.

It's good to question why we're here on planet Earth. What's not good is to live with that feeling that we're nothing more than a skin-covered skeleton. Because we're far, far more.

Your brain, for example, consumes 20% of your body's energy. It's working even when you're resting, constantly thinking and creating. During the night it helps to solve problems through the medium of dreams (if you remember them, write your dreams down and see what kinds of themes come up). This organ inside your skull is used for far more than retaining information. Sometimes it breaks down, which is why we're here.

The human brain can do far more than we give it credit for. It's often said that we know about outer space than what the brain can do. Your brain is what allows you to form your thoughts, personal opinions, ideas, and to experience and react to the world around you. We're not zombies. We don't just wander mindlessly from one place to another. We are able to think, feel, and process the world around us in a way that a zombie wouldn't.

You're constantly producing energy and you'll be able to pick up on the energy around you (often called "the sixth sense", "gut instinct", or "intuition"). You know when a situation is right or wrong. You know when a person is someone that you'd like to deal with as opposed to someone you want to keep away from. For a moment close your eyes and feel the world around you. What do you feel? What do you see? How does the person on the other side of the room feel to you?

You're not here just to exist. You're here to produce, travel, create, love, and so much more. You're not here to just take pills and sleep. You're here to stand up for what you believe in, to sing, to draw, to dance, to speak. You're not here to just be a name on a medical list. You're here to be a unique and beautiful person no matter what life has thrown at you. You're not here just to work from nine to five for forty years of your life. You're here to find your voice and use it in a way that will benefit you and the world around you.

You are far more than a skin-covered skeleton. You are far more than your diagnosis and the medication you take. You are far more than a repetitive job. You are here to be beautiful and to show the world that there is no stigma to the person you are. We only have a finite amount of time on this planet so make it count.

BELIEVE

Believe. One little word that, for so many people, holds a myriad of emotions. Believing in yourself, believing in your partner, believing in the words that are written on a page; all are phrases that can be hard to process.

Believing in yourself can be hard. We become so worn down with whatever our brain is doing that thinking, or doing, anything else can add strain to our already tired bodies. Yet we know that we're on this planet for something far more than a routine daily existence. We know that we have stories to tell, places to go and visit, and dreams to live out. But whatever is happening to us physically and mentally can drain us of the energy that we need to even begin doing everything else.

The world around us also has a tendency to beat us down. Daily we're shown images of people whose lives are far better than ours may ever be. We're almost forced to look at the lives of celebrities and compare ourselves to them. *We'll never be like them. We'll never have their lives. We'll never have what they have.* These become our mantras and, time and again, we find ourselves pushed back in to the little box that has been created around us, and any belief that we had in ourselves is slowly stripped away.

I never used to believe in myself. No matter how many people told me that they loved my writing, I still didn't believe them, or myself. For a long time I hated my writing style. I thought that it was too simplistic and didn't carry the weight that I wanted it to.

It took many years before I realised that I was writing in the style that I needed. Nothing could change that. The words I was putting on to paper and the way that they were being structured was one that many people could understand. I didn't have to use long words or complicated sentences. I just had to be me.

My self belief has been eroded throughout my life. This chipping away at my confidence started in school and went on through college and university. Over and over I was told that I wouldn't amount to anything and that my ideas were useless. I didn't receive the support that I needed, ruining my confidence and self esteem along the way. I learned to keep quiet, keeping my thoughts to myself. Because why say something when you're only going to be bullied for it?

I still have moments of doubt. There are still times when I don't quite believe in myself and my unique abilities. But I'm getting better at it. Every day is a new day, a day to change myself for the better and strengthen my belief in myself.

Whether you've been beaten down or just lack the self confidence to do what you want to do, you can change your mind and believe.

You can believe in yourself. You can do whatever your heart is telling you to do. You have to learn to tune out the noise that surrounds us. Turn off the TV. Log out of social media. Don't look at the glossy magazines on the news-stand. Drown out friends who gossip about others.

In the chapter "Personal Affirmations" you'll find four very important words. *I believe in myself.* Say them as often as you need to. Say them until you feel the love and warmth grow inside of you. Say them until you feel strong enough to go out in to the world to do your thing. Say them even as you go about doing what you.

THE COMING OF SPRING

Spring is a beautiful time of the year. The days get longer and the weather becomes warmer as the world eases its way out of another winter. Around us plants and flowers begin to grow again, new leaves and petals unfurling from branches and stems. Parks and gardens become a riot of colour and we begin to feel better.

This new season can also be seen as a time for ourselves to be reborn. Often we struggle with ourselves. We see ourselves as unchangeable, as people who must stay the same from one day to the next. We carry baggage from years previously, refusing to let it go because it's the only thing we know. That baggage, whether its the ghosts of past relationships or the hooks of a previous job that have become buried beneath our skin, feels like it defines us. It feels like that's all that we have to offer to the world and that nothing we can do will change that.

But, like the flowers that are starting to sprout, we too can decide to shed the darkness of winter and leave our old lives behind. We can become new people, reborn in to a brand new world.

There are so many quotes that relate to this evolution:

Every day is a new day.

Every day is a new chapter.

Every day is a chance to start over.

Every morning starts with a new page.

Each morning we are born again.

That's because every day is a chance to start over. It's a chance to shed the skin of the person that you once were and become the person that you want to be. You're not confined by your job title, relationship status, social media profile, or medical issues. You are a person who can choose to change their life. Your life probably won't change over night but, like the coming of spring, you go through the slow process of changing a little something every day. Finally, at some point in the future, you will find yourself in the place that you want to be.

Don't allow yourself to become inhibited by the person you believe that you are (or the person that you believe you should be). Don't allow yourself to be imprisoned by the thinking of others whether that's friends, family, or the media. Don't allow yourself to believe what people tell you about living your life. Most importantly, don't give up, no matter how hard the process may seem.

Instead, allow yourself to grow and flourish. Let the petals of your life uncurl and live your life your way.

TRUST YOUR JOURNEY

"I am learning to trust the journey even when I do not understand it." - Mila Bron

Does your heart ache with the need to do something? Maybe you want to write, paint, travel, care for the sick, or move house. You want to follow what your heart is telling you but maybe the daily grind gets in the way. Maybe you're scared or stuck in a rut or don't know where to start.

Take a deep breath and start from the beginning. Make a list of what you'd really love to do with your life. Want to live on an island? Put it on there. Want to buy your own house? Put it on there. Write down everything that you want to do, look it over and decide which ones you can feasibly achieve in the here and now.

Perhaps one of your dreams is to write a novel. Do you have an idea for a story? If so, make a little time in your life to start working on it, even if it's only five or ten minutes every other day. Go to bed a little earlier and lie in bed with a notebook. Set the TV to record that show you want to watch. Put the cleaning off for another day. Turn your phone off. Every little thing you do to free up time to do what you want to do is a step in the right direction. You may not see the results straight away but you're getting there, one step at a time.

Doing something new is about commitment and being true to yourself. For a long time, I wrote nothing but fiction and I loved every moment of it. Over the past year, that desire has waned and been replaced with the need to write non-fiction. I still dabble in working on my novels but the drive to finish anything has dwindled. The last thing I completed was the novel/screenplay combo *Dance in the Rain* back in 2014.

To prepare for a new phase in my life I knew that I needed to change some of my skills. So I started brushing up on my research skills. I also started running interviews on my website. Whenever I was offered a guest blog or the chance to speak somewhere, I took it. I asked myself, "Can I sit and listen and give someone my entire focus for the length of an interview?". For me, that can be extremely difficult so it's something I've been practising with family, friends, and work colleagues. Now I'm hopefully putting the final pieces of the puzzle together in order to start this brand new chapter.

Changing your life doesn't happen overnight but it can be done. You have to be true to yourself. If that yearning for something new is living in you, take time to think about what you want to do and how you can get there. It might not happen today. It might not happen next month. But you can do it. You can do whatever you put your mind to.

BREAK IT DOWN

Living with mental health issues can make even the smallest task an unbearable chore. Need to get out of bed? Forget it. Want to go to the supermarket? You'd rather not, thanks. Had an invitation to a party? A night of Netflix seems like a better option. But if you could do anything, without the fear of judgement, what would you do?

I've always wanted to be a writer. Deep down, I know that it's what I'm called to do. But writing an entire book can be a daunting task. Where do you start? How do you develop your characters? Can you sustain the enthusiasm and story for months, even years, until you've finished it?

I started by writing short 100 word stories for a writing website. They were small, compact scenes designed to show a brief moment in time. Gradually, they became longer until eventually I found myself with an entire novel (*Mars on the Rise*). I've now written several books, numerous short stories, screenplays, treatments, interviews, and everything in between.

Something else that took time working towards involved the trip of a lifetime. In 2004, I wanted to visit Las Vegas. I had it all planned out, right down to staying at the Luxor hotel. But, at the time, I had no money and didn't have the confidence to go alone.

In 2013, I met someone who takes annual vacations to Las Vegas. She invited me to go with them. Yet there were several problems to overcome. I still didn't have a lot of money (albeit more than I had in 2004), I live several thousand miles from Las Vegas, and I hadn't travelled long haul by myself for over a decade.

The solution? To fund the trip, I applied for, and received, a 0% credit card. Over the next year I paid the holiday off a little at a time. Knowing that there was someone who would meet me at the other end soothed the stressful feelings of travelling alone and I solved my fear of travelling so far by myself by making sure that I was thoroughly prepared. This included having valid travel insurance, studying airport maps, and having a phone that was compatible with US networks.

Las Vegas was everything that I ever imagined it would be and it got me back in to the swing of travelling after a decade of not doing so.

One of the best ways to achieve any task is to break it down in to smaller pieces. You don't have to do everything in one go. If cooking a meal looks like a mountain, think about how it can be made into simpler tasks and then make a step-by-step list of what you need to do. Work through the list at your own pace and you'll eventually find yourself achieving whatever you want to achieve.

HELP YOURSELF

There's only one person on this planet who can help you.

You.

You are the only person who can make the decision with what to do with your life. You are the only person who can make the decision on where to go, what to see, and how to live. If you want to get treatment for yourself, that's your decision. If you want to travel, that's your decision. If you want to work, that's your decision

But the only person who will help you get to where you want to go, whether that's a physical or mental destination, is you. Of course, you can ask for help along the way but no one is going to come up to you and offer it all on a plate. You have to get out there and work for what you want, be that better health, a better job, a better home, or a better life.

I had to learn that and I learned it the hard way. I believe that the things I wanted in life would fall in to my lap. I believed that I didn't have to work to get somewhere and that just daydreaming about the life I wanted would be enough.

Boy, was I wrong.

Over the past several years, I've had quite a few doses of reality be it from issues flaring up at work to tough love from family to trying to open career doors that aren't yet ready to be opened. Each time has been a painful learning experience and I've learned to stop and evaluate my life. What do I want? How can I get there? Do I need new skills to achieve it? How can I get out of the rut that I'm stuck in? How could I change myself to become a better person?

Because of these experiences, I decided to move away from writing fiction and turn to non-fiction. I realised that I had a talent for getting people to talk and to being able to listen to what they had to say. I decided to combine that with my writing and began working on two books that documented the lives of the people around me. As I started working on the books, I realised that I was the happiest I'd been. No longer did I feel stressed. Nor did I feel like I was pushing at doors that were locked.

If there's something that you want to do, only you can get there. You need to sit back and evaluate your life. Do you notice patterns of conflict in your life? If so, how can you solve them? What do you need to change about yourself? Are you too critical? Does your anger flare too quickly? Do you need to gain new skills? Do you need to move house? Do you need to change your career path? Do you need to stop hanging out with certain people?

Keep a journal and see what pushes your buttons. You don't have to write in it every day and, over time, you'll be able to begin working on getting to the place that you want to be.

You can do whatever you put your mind to but, in order to get there, you need to give yourself a dose of tough love in order to get there.

Happiness isn't a destination; it's a journey.

EMPOWER EACH OTHER

We live in a world where people are encouraged to tear one another down. They're told that, in order to get ahead in life, they have to tread on other peoples dreams and berate one another. If it's not a dream they're taking apart, it's another person's body. Or their personality. Or their style of dress. We live in a world that is polluted by hostility to those around us. We're conditioned to be constantly on guard and to have an explanation for every second of our lives. We're watched and judged, not by the government, but by one another.

What if we could flip that around and, instead of beating each other up, we could empower one another? Wouldn't it be nice to live in a world where, instead of climbing over each other to reach the top, we could climb it hand in hand?

It's time to empower one another. It's time to take back control of ourselves and who we are, to live our lives in a beautiful and productive way. It's time for us to look at one another as friends rather than enemies. It's time for us to love ourselves and those around us.

We can make a difference in one another's lives. We can choose to step away from the crowds and be different. We can choose to be loving and compassionate. We can help one another along this journey called life.

But how?

- Find something good to say about someone's work. They've probably had it picked apart by different people and your compliment could change how they feel about what they're doing. Encourage one another and lift people up. You could change a person's life.
- Climb the ladders together and love those who've supported you along the way. Say thank you and give out hugs. The way you treat a person is your trademark.
- Stay strong together. There's people out there whose life mission is to make everyone else feel bad. When they come along, rally together and encourage one another to keep going. The road may feel long but the people you're with can turn the journey in to a festival.
- Get excited about each other's lives. Does someone have a big project going? Is there a new band that needs a little love? Share them on social media and celebrate both the big, and small, achievements together.
- Make like-minded friends along the way. Your tribe always has room for one more. Welcome them with open arms.

Life is supposed to be fun and we're supposed to love one another. Make sure yours is a party that has an open invitation and is a party that none of you will ever forget.

STEP IN TO THE LIGHT

Light visualisations have been used for many years to help people protect themselves against the harsh world that they live in. Many people find them to be a useful tool when dealing with the day to day stresses of life.

Getting Rid of Negativity

Sit or stand with your feet firmly planted on the floor. Picture a shaft of bright white light entering the crown of your head and travelling down your spine before exiting in to the earth. See the black fragments of negativity leaving your body and feel the warmth of the light fill you.

Protecting Yourself

With mental health issues, you're often more sensitive to those around you. Criticism and complaints as well as negative atmospheres such as work places and family gatherings can hurt far more when you're at your lowest and most vulnerable. Unfortunately we can't always stay in the safety of our own personal space. But you can create one for when you're out and about.

Again, sit or stand with your feet on the ground. Visualise a sphere of white light surrounding you. The sphere extends for several feet all around you, enclosing you in a safe space. Whenever you feel the need to strengthen it, picture the sphere becoming bigger and brighter.

Your Armour

As mentioned before, you may find yourself going in to a situation that you find stressful. This may be a work place, a family gathering, a medical appointment, or any number of different places.

As well as your sphere of light, you can also visualise yourself wearing a suit of armour. Picture the different pieces being added to your body including the helmet to protect your mind and the breast plate to protect your heart and soul. For added protection, see yourself carrying a shield to deflect any negative energy or words. Know that you are protecting the parts of yourself that are the most vulnerable, including your spirit.

BE GRATEFUL

Being thankful for the things in our life is a great way to help alleviate the darkness in our minds. Having a grateful mind helps to change the negativity that we feel in to positivity. When practised on a daily basis, gratitude can literally help to rewire our brains.

Saying thank you is how I helped myself out of the depths of depression. I thanked the world for the lessons it set, no matter how painful they were. I said thank you to my friends and family for the things they did for me. I was grateful for the food on my table, the roof over my head, or the ability to get up and live another day.

Over time I noticed that my mind was more inclined to be happy. I scowled less and smiled more. I felt lighter and when I slipped back in to negative thought patterns, I noticed how much heavier my body felt. Being grateful soon came naturally and I was saying thank you for everything.

Being grateful can seem like a chore when our mental health is low. Our brains are automatically set in to survival mode and all we want to do is make it through the day.

It isn't hard to be thankful for one thing every day. You may love the sun; say thank you when the sun is out. You may enjoy your favourite meal; say thank you when you have it. Your bed may be warm and comfortable; say thank you for the safe sanctuary you can fall in to at the end of the day.

You don't have to say thank you out loud nor in the presence of other people. You can write down what you feel thankful for. Keep a Gratitude Journal where you list one (or more) things every day that you appreciate having in your life. It may be the people in your life, or that you have clothes on your back, or that you get to wake up every day. You may be thankful for having a roof over your head, for dancing in the rain, or for hearing your favourite song.

Be thankful once a way and, over time, you'll feel yourself become happier and lighter. As the darkness recedes, you'll find that you're grateful for more than you could ever imagine. And, along the way, you're also giving yourself the tools to help with your mental health. Whenever the darkness begins to return (as it inevitably does), look back over the lists of things you've said thank you for. Your heart will be warmed by all that you've been through and will remind you to keep taking life one day at a time.

The thankful heart opens our eyes to a multitude of blessings that continually surrounds us.
- James E. Faust

LIFE LESSONS FROM LIL' BUB

Have you met Lil' Bub? She's a tiny four pound cat who overcame all the odds to become who she is today. At a year old, Bub was diagnosed with osteopetrosis and her owner was informed that it was only a matter of time before she became immobile. Yet Bub defied all the odds and a video posted in September 2014 shows her unwavering determination and amazing recovery.

As well as being a space traveller, musician, You Tube star, and advocate for adopting pets from shelters, Bub has a special message to share with the planet. It's a message of positivity, acceptance, and to provide inspiration around the world by proving that being different is something to be proud of.

So what can we learn from Bub?

- What would you do if you knew you couldn't fail? Would you climb mountains? Make movies? Trek to the North Pole? All to often we don't want to anything new because we fear failure. Don't believe that anything you do is doomed from the start. Follow your heart and see where it leads you.
- Keep on going even if it seems like the battle is never-ending. Life gets tough. Life gets painful. But they're all experiences we can learn from. Take those unhappy moments and use them to build the life you want.

- Never give up. The finish line may seem like a million miles away. But it gets closer with all that you do and with every passing day. Be determined and keep going. Rome wasn't built in a day.
- Find your passion and walk, run, jump, or waddle with it. Love it with all your heart and embrace it as your own. It's not about making money or being famous. It's about finding that one thing that makes you smile every time you think about it.
- Be confident, even if you think you can't. It'll get you a long way.
- Positive mental attitude. Start every day thinking it's going to be the best day ever. Because you never know what's going to happen!
- Be the light. Even if everyone around you is full of negativity and drama, be the one who makes them smile.
- Happiness isn't a destination, it's a journey.
- Spread a little love, magic, and positivity along the way!

LAUGHTER IS THE BEST MEDICINE

This morning I've done nothing but laugh. I laughed at the funny photo that a friend had sent, then at the cat videos on Facebook, and finally at the Reddit posts. My Mum made me laugh with a random comment. My Dad made me laugh with his reaction to a news story.

Laughter really is good for the soul. It stimulates the production of the happy hormone, serotonin, making us feel good in the process. Studies have shown that laughter can help with everything from alleviating stress to stimulating your heart and lungs to soothing tension. It's the body's natural way of helping to clear out so much of what we experience on a daily basis.

For some people, laughing can be hard. But there are many ways of finding something that will tickle your funny bone. Seeing the funny side of life is a start. Tripped over the cat this morning? Laugh about it. Put mayonnaise instead of milk in to your tea? Cry tears of laughter instead.

Finding a favourite comedian is another way to get those feel good hormones bouncing. The internet allows us to go looking for whatever tickles our fancy. Maybe there's a comedy sketch you remember from years ago or a film that had you rolling in the aisles. You may not remember the title but it's guaranteed that you'll find something along the way that will make your sides ache from laughing.

There are songs that are written with the primary purpose of making us laugh. Again, start with the musicians you do now and keep looking until you find something that makes you smile.

It can only take a matter of moments to find a website that's dedicated to making us laugh. Memes, funny videos, and photos that will make us giggle are all out there, waiting to be discovered by us.

Books are another source of humorous entertainment and your local book store will probably have a section dedicated to them. There are books covering all kinds of life events from parenting to owning a cat to going to work.

Laughter therapy is an exercise that's becoming popular and is based on the belief that voluntary laughter produces the same physiological and psychological results as spontaneous laughter does. There are many practitioners and classes around the world and a quick internet search should throw up ones that are local to you.

So laugh. Laugh long and loud. Laugh until your ribs ache and tears are rolling down your cheeks. Laugh until you feel good, because you deserve all the happiness that the world has to offer.

YOU ARE UNIQUE

There is no one else like you on the planet. No one else will have the same fingerprints, same body shape, same eyes, same laugh, same smile. No one else who came before you or who comes after you will be the same as you are right now. The mould was well and truly broken after you were created.

No one else sees the world as you do. No one else experiences life in the way that you do. No one else can express themselves in the way that you. No one else is as wonderfully and perfectly created as you are.

List three unique things that you love about yourself. This could be anything from your hair colour to your handwriting to your ability to show empathy. There are no right or wrong answers because this is about you, and you alone.

1.

2.

3.

YOU ARE NOT ALONE

You are not alone on this journey.

We walk with you, together as one, supporting and loving one another through the good days, and the bad.

We embrace you and welcome you home, taking away your fear and replacing it with hope.

No longer will you be alone, nor will you face this by yourself. There will be others around you, holding and helping you, sharing their experiences with you as you walk this path.

You may feel alone but you are not. Look up, open you eyes, and see the people who surround you. They smile and open their arms, holding you close as they reassure you that life will not always be this hard, or this painful, or this dark.

We are with you, in person and in spirit, reassuring you and helping you to grow your wings. We will love you, nurture you, and accept you just the way you are.

You are not alone.

You are loved.

Live. Love. Laugh.

THE FEEL-GOOD LISTS

Films and songs to help pick you up and keep you going.

FEEL-GOOD PLAYLIST

You Make Me Feel (Mighty Real) – Sylvester

The Day Brings – Brad

Learn to Fly – Foo Fighters

What a Beautiful Day – Levellers

Tarzan Boy – Baltimora

Happy – Pharrell Williams

Raise Your Glass – Pink

Steal My Sunshine – Len

All Star – Smash Mouth

Pump It Up – Elvis Costello

Born This Way – Lady Gaga

Giorgio by Moroder – Daft Punk

Oh Lori – Alessi Brothers

Well Run Dry – Phat Phunktion

More Than a Feeling – Boston

The Spirit of Radio – Rush

Freedom 90 – George Michael

Mr Blue Sky – ELO

Valentine – The Delays

Everybody Loves You - Sigue Sigue Sputnik

Echo Beach – Martha and the Muffins

I'm Alright – Jo Dee Messina

Hawaiian Rollercoaster Ride – Lilo and Stitch

Clearly Now The Rain Has Gone – Hothouse Flowers

Bridge Over Troubled Water – Simon & Garfunkel

Hump De Bump – Red Hot Chili Peppers

Everybody's Free (To Wear Sunscreen) – Baz Luhrmann

FEEL-GOOD FILMS

Empire Records

Practical Magic

Pretty in Pink

Grease 2

The Princess Bride

Back to the Future

Hocus Pocus

Shaun of the Dead

Mannequin

Dirty Dancing

Dragonfly

Mary Poppins

Forrest Gump

Enchanted

Big

The 5th Element

Muppets Christmas Carol

Lilo and Stitch

ABOUT THE AUTHOR

Rachael lives in the heart of England and, when she's not writing, she enjoys listening to music, walking, photography, and UFOlogy. Her view is that life is a journey and that every day is a blank page just waiting to be written upon.

www.raegee.co.uk
Instagram: @RoswellPublishing
Twitter: @VeetuIndustries
facebook.com/thequeenofsteam

Made in the USA
Las Vegas, NV
07 September 2021

29780811R00083